THE SCIENCE OF
PLANETARY
SIGNATURES
IN MEDICINE

"Jennifer Gehl takes us on a tour through history. Visiting a wide variety of cultures, systems, philosophers, and thinkers, an underlying thread is unmistakable. We are connected to *all* of nature, including and especially, the planetary energies of our solar system. Astrology can and does play a central role in all of life, including the healing arts. In *The Science of Planetary Signatures in Medicine,* we have the basic premise elucidated with striking clarity: There is an order to the universe. What we do with this realization is up to us. How might we integrate astrology and nature's intelligence into 21st-century healing arts? That is the task before us, and this book is an excellent guide for all of us."

ERIC MEYERS, AUTHOR OF *THE ASTROLOGY OF AWAKENING*

"*The Science of Planetary Signatures in Medicine* will surprise you as a comprehensive and beautifully written text. It offers a strong measure of historical and scientific background while remaining crystal clear and intriguing. Gehl embraces the beauty of music as she draws out the mathematical roots of music theory and lays out its integral connection to the planet and universal laws at play. As an example, we get to explore with the author how the principles of harmonics in music apply to other vibratory phenomena in the universe. The book is a lucid, scholastic exploration that every practitioner will want and will use. It will be hard not to devour every concept on the first read . . . it will continue to serve as an excellent, authoritative reference for years to come!"

STEVEN WEISS, MS, DC, RYT, AUTHOR OF
THE INJURY-FREE YOGA PRACTICE

"Jennifer Gehl synthesizes cosmology, history, philosophy, mathematics, music, and physics. She applies these perspectives in a way that expands our knowledge of these disciplines in relationship to healing. Ultimately the connection between sound healing and physics is presented. Healers of all disciplines, and particularly Acutonics practitioners, will find connections that develop the conversation surrounding many of the principles involved in healing."

WILLIAM MORRIS, PH.D., DAOM, L.AC., AUTHOR OF
*TRANSFORMATION: TREATING TRAUMA WITH
ACUPUNCTURE AND HERBS*

THE SCIENCE OF
PLANETARY SIGNATURES IN MEDICINE

Restoring the Cosmic Foundations of Healing

JENNIFER T. GEHL, MHS
WITH Marc S. Micozzi, M.D., Ph.D.

Healing Arts Press
Rochester, Vermont • Toronto, Canada

Healing Arts Press
One Park Street
Rochester, Vermont 05767
www.HealingArtsPress.com

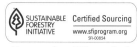

Text stock is SFI certified

Healing Arts Press is a division of Inner Traditions International

Note to the reader: This book is intended as an informational guide. The remedies, approaches, and techniques described herein are meant to supplement, and not to be a substitute for, professional medical care or treatment. They should not be used to treat a serious ailment without prior consultation with a qualified health care professional.

Library of Congress Cataloging-in-Publication Data
Names: Gehl, Jennifer T., author. | Micozzi, Marc S., 1953– author.
Title: The science of planetary signatures in medicine : restoring the cosmic foundations of healing / Jennifer T. Gehl with Marc S. Micozzi.
Description: Rochester, Vermont : Healing Arts Press, [2017] | Includes bibliographical references and index.
Identifiers: LCCN 2016021010 (print) | LCCN 2016021947 (e-book) | ISBN 9781620554982 (pbk.) | ISBN 9781620554999 (e-book)
Subjects: | MESH: Holistic Health | Metaphysics | Mythology | Yin-Yang | Naturopathy | Spiritual Therapies
Classification: LCC R733 (print) | LCC R733 (e-book) | NLM W 61 | DDC 615.5—dc23
LC record available at https://lccn.loc.gov/2016021010

Printed and bound in the United States by Lake Book Manufacturing, Inc.
The text stock is SFI certified. The Sustainable Forestry Initiative® program promotes sustainable forest management.

10 9 8 7 6 5 4 3 2 1

Text design by Virginia Scott Bowman and layout by Debbie Glogover
This book was typeset in Garamond Premier Pro with Hypatia Sans, Futura, Gill Sans and Avenir.

To send correspondence to the authors of this book, mail a first-class letter to the authors c/o Inner Traditions • Bear & Company, One Park Street, Rochester, VT 05767, and we will forward the communication, or contact the authors directly at **www.soundworksbygehl.com** or **soundworksbygehl@gmail.com** for Jennifer Gehl and **www.drmicozzi.com** for Marc Micozzi.

This book is dedicated to all souls whose ancient self already knows what is written on and in between these pages, but may have forgotten. When darkness seems to divide us, there is a light inextinguishable guiding us back to connection, and a voice that calls us ever toward harmony.

Mankind needs less to be instructed than to be reminded.

SAMUEL JOHNSON,
SEVENTEENTH-CENTURY ENGLISH PHILOSOPHER

CONTENTS

ACKNOWLEDGMENTS

I extend profound gratitude to Jon Graham, and the entire editing team at Inner Traditions International (ITI), for providing me with expert assistance, invaluable support, and above all, the opportunity to publish this work. Sincere thanks to Donna Carey, L.Ac, and Ellen F. Franklin, Ph.D., today's natural scientists and pioneers, without whose research, support, and editorial assistance this work would not exist.

To my mother JoEllen, and my recently deceased father, Ken (1933–2015), I owe a debt of gratitude for the generosity and love that has always guided and supported me while navigating life's difficult passages; and to all my family members, whose worldview, while different from mine, has always been motivated by love.

To the many friends, colleagues, and mentors—that host of "silent pioneers"—whose influence continues to inspire me to seek new pathways of understanding, and given me the courage to express a new (ancient) worldview, you are cherished beyond words. Most importantly, I want to thank the silent host from the "other side" who have unceasingly loved, patiently guided, profoundly inspired, and secretly indoctrinated me into a world of unimaginable beauty and heavenly harmony.

J.T.G

FOREWORD

Is it not . . . plausible that human nature, in all its creative multidimensional depths and heights, emerges from the very essence of the cosmos, and that the human spirit is the spirit of the cosmos itself . . . ?

RICHARD TARNAS, *COSMOS AND PSYCHE*

The Science of Planetary Signatures in Medicine is a rich, multilayered exploration of the direct connections among the planets, their movements in the heavens, and their impacts on human health. This book explores the wisdom of the ancients and traces patterns of correspondences from prehistory to modern science.

Herein the inner cosmos is represented as a replica of the outer cosmos and strong evidence for the affinities between the microcosm (physical body) and the macrocosm (universe) is presented. Our cells reflect the images of the galaxies and the universe. When we explore the vast and intricate cosmos—galaxies, planets, organisms, organs, cells, molecules, and atoms—there indeed appears a fundamental order, or fundamental essence, that corresponds to (or at the very least hints at) the principle of harmony and the music of the spheres. Although planetary gods are not playing the strings of the universe, our ancestors' insights and intuitions about the relations of humanity to the vast universe that surrounded them was correct. When humanity is seen as a microcosm reflecting the macrocosm of the heavens—"As above, so below" and "As without, so within"—we understand, as if for the very first time, the meaning behind this ancient adage.

Whatever paradigms or beliefs you hold with regard to religion, science, allopathic medicine, integrative medicine, energy healing, and/or astrology, or whether you are simply seeking wisdom, a key for advancement and evolution is to keep an open mind and heart. The health care model is changing rapidly as people in record numbers continue to seek what has been labeled Complementary and Alternative Medicine (CAM). In the healing modalities represented by CAM there is a recognition that health is a dynamic state of balance that requires shifts, adaptations, and recovery in a person-centered approach to well-being that moves away from the materialist model separating mind and body and the reductionism that breaks everything down into its smallest component parts.

Various theories in physics and cosmology, such as renowned physicist David Bohm's exploration of wholeness and the implicate order, attempt to demonstrate that the workings and transformations of the parts affect the whole and are able to both order and organize nonlinear functions through a process of enfoldment. Essentially there are subtle forces at work that interact, organize, and affect the larger picture on all levels (not unlike the theories put forth regarding the macrocosm and the microcosm, or which are implicit in the tenets of East Asian cosmology and medicine). Bohm was trying to reconcile Einstein's theory of relativity and quantum theory while accounting for nonlocal effects, which posit that nothing is complete in and of itself. There is mutual participation (entanglement) of everything with everything and Bohm clearly articulates that everything that falls under the purview of "science" cannot be practiced in a fragmentary way as independent parts but must be explored through an awareness of the undivided wholeness of the universe.

Unfortunately, the modern focus of academic research continues to be dominated by those "splitters" who seek to demonstrate differences rather than similarities, to break down and tear apart rather than look for commonalities and the potential for cross-disciplinary collaboration. In the unending quest for more medical research funding we see double-blind studies and control groups that rarely take into consideration the whole person and the quality of life changes they might experience if their illness or condition was seen from a physical, emotional, and/or spiritual perspective. Despite the growth in qualitative research we often fail to value the subjective quality of life experiences, and believe that the "objectivity" of logical positivism is the Holy Grail.

In medicine, there is the "if not this, that; if not that, this" approach to differential diagnosis that invalidates anamnesis, the ability to remember and reflect on (or simply not forget) previous foundations that contribute to the whole. It is rare to be able to take a holistic approach to any research or education, to be able to step back and examine studies across multiple fields or specialties when framing new studies or the acquisition of knowledge. Jennifer Gehl has done just that. She has effectively woven together research findings that span thousands of years and diverse traditions from the disciplines of early medicine, mathematics, myths and legends, sacred geometry, music, and East Asian medicine. She provides compelling perspectives as to why we should care about the influences of the planets and the cosmos on life on Earth.

We first met Jennifer in 2004 when she came to an Acutonics class in Loveland, Colorado. Acutonics is a healing modality that uses planetary tones on the meridian system of the body as well as on its acupuncture points. This class was an unusually large, advanced group of health care practitioners, including nurses, acupuncturists, bodywork practitioners, and physicians. Many of these students would go on to become certified Acutonics practitioners and teachers. Jennifer was one of those exceptional pupils: a seeker of knowledge who attended the intensive course with a desire to deepen her understanding of the powerful connections that exist among music, astrology, and Chinese medicine, all of which are explored in our program. She was an active contributor in class and possessed a profound understanding of planetary influences on human health. She went on to complete her studies to become certified as both an Acutonics practitioner and teacher, and she also developed a course in the basics of astrological medicine, which is now offered as an elective in our program.

Her continued quest for knowledge led her to pursue her master's degree in health sciences, and to seek out Dr. Marc S. Micozzi, the visionary anthropologist medical doctor responsible for the seminal text-book *Fundamentals of Complementary and Alternative Medicine*, which is now going into its sixth edition. This connection resulted in Jennifer being asked to contribute a piece on Acutonics to the textbook. She describes how Acutonics blends ancient wisdom, East Asian medicine, archetypes, myths, and modern science into a cohesive approach to health and holism that incorporates the use of vibratory energy, or sound, of the planets on acupuncture points. Jennifer then felt compelled to research and write a far more comprehensive work that weaves together ancient wisdom and modern science to provide a fresh perspective on how this knowledge can be used to redefine our approach to health and holism. She was encouraged to pursue this path by Dr. Micozzi, who offered his wisdom, years of writing experience, and editorial guidance.

Whatever name you use—mind-body medicine, integrative medi-cine, or CAM—the underlying principle of this discipline is a holis-tic approach to medicine and health care that focuses on the whole person. These include the physical, mental, emotional, and spiritual/energetic aspects of the individual. This approach is distinct from what has come to be identified as Western or allopathic medicine, which is primarily focused on the individual parts of the body such as organs, tissues, and cells, and which has viewed the mind as separate from the body. Jennifer provides us with a way to think about mind-body medi-cine and to more deeply understand the influences of the cosmos on human health. She defines this new perspective on health and healing as authentic medicine.

Several concepts explored by Jennifer are also employed in Acutonics and in some practices of Oriental medicine, which include the five phase, or five element, theory, built on the assumption that the forces that exist in the cycles of nature and that occur in the outside world are duplicated within our bodies at every level. Five phase theories are built on correspondences in which the person is seen as a small universe reflecting the greater universe. When elements coexist in balance and harmony the person is in good health, however, when physiological and psychological processes are out of balance, they must be readjusted or illness sets in. Moving with the cycles of nature results in a full and harmonious life; if there is imbalance, mental and physical health suffers. Jennifer provides us with a depth of knowledge and understanding that invites us to explore the value inherent in these healing traditions and to recognize their place in the future practice of medicine.

The Science of Planetary Signatures in Medicine is an invitation to healing and hope. This book opens a door into how we might embrace ancient wisdom with the best of modern science and truly return art and spirit to medicine. It helps rediscover the spirit of our ancient teachers and the artistic and creative approach that many early physicians employed—one that many contemporary medical practitioners are beginning to embrace. It promotes partnerships with our patients, and invites us to support their personal journeys as they take an active role in their path to health and holism. It requires courage to be open to the infinite potential of the universe, to release limiting thoughts, and to recognize that we are all part of an infinite web and have access to miracles that defy current science.

ELLEN F. FRANKLIN, PH.D., AND DONNA CAREY, M.S., L.AC.
ACUTONICS INSTITUTE OF INTEGRATIVE MEDICINE
LLANO, NEW MEXICO

ELLEN F. FRANKLIN, PH.D., is cofounder and CEO of the Acutonics Institute of Integrative Medicine. For more than fifteen years she has been involved in the development and dissemination of educational programs in vibrational sound therapy rooted in Oriental Medicine and psychology. Ellen is a coauthor of *Acutonics from Galaxies to Cells: Planetary Science, Harmony and Medicine,* a 2012 gold medal recipient in the Independent Publishing Awards.

DONNA CAREY is cofounder of the Acutonics Institute of Integrative Medicine and vice president of Devachan Press. She is a licensed acupuncturist, herbalist, sound healer, educator, and poet, trained in Western and Eastern medicine and the arts. Donna is coauthor of *Acutonics: There's No Place Like Ohm— Sound Healing, Oriental Medicine and the Cosmic Mysteries* and *Acutonics from Galaxies to Cells: Planetary Science, Harmony and Medicine.*

PREFACE

By Jennifer T. Gehl, MHS

Dear Reader,

As you embark on the journey this book has to offer, I invite you to keep an open mind. Inasmuch as it will reveal itself to you, it has revealed itself to me, chapter by chapter, through an engaging, awe-inspiring, world of magic that wants to come through at this time. The path leading to this book's publication was strewn with surprising synchronicities, inspiring gratitude and trust in the "implicate order." At the same time, this experience has been humbling. Along the way, I had to make adjustments concerning long-held beliefs about Earth's history, and stay open to revising what I thought I already knew.

I would be remiss to represent myself as a voice of authority on the ideas presented here, and that is not my goal. It has been my goal to simply allow new information to reveal itself in a manner that supports growth and healing, while weaving together the threads from our ancient past with a more current paradigm. The only thing one can ever know with certainty is what is experienced personally, and I would characterize my personal experience while writing this book as one of catharsis.

No matter how much knowledge a person acquires, there can be no wisdom (or true healing) without applying that knowledge to one's life. For those with worldly views supported by worldly experiences, the information contained in these pages may not resonate. My journey has not included being a world traveler, archaeologist, historian, scientist, physician, philosopher, or spiritual guru. On the other hand, it has been an inner journey of cultivating trust in my own experiences, even when those experiences have felt like utter failure or completely strayed from mainstream thought.

Along the way, there were plenty of times when I tried to impose "my truth"—according to the experience I was having at the time—on other people, only to discover the disappointment of resistance. Real truth can only come from a *personal* process of discovery. More importantly, it can only be *experienced* through the process of *discovering the Self*. And for each one of us, that looks and feels a little bit different, similar to variations on a theme.

As for my process of self-discovery, what has shaped my experiences comes from inner, "otherworldly," and spiritual (celestial) encounters that began when I was very young. These encounters have fostered me throughout my life. I have always felt the presence of unseen helpers who light my path, guide my steps, and provide a sense of safety and security to me. Offered now is a brief synopsis of the "outer" journey that has led me to this point.

SYNTHESIZING MUSIC, ASTROLOGY, AND CHINESE MEDICINE

At the age of six, I began to study music, first with the piano, and a year later with the violin. Raised in a loving, supportive, and devoutly Catholic family, I practiced music and Catholicism without question. Although I had mystical encounters and experiences, I lacked faith and confidence in my own abilities in these areas until I encountered astrology as a teenager.

Astrology gave me something that no other doctrine provided: the real, applicable, evidence of an infinite intelligence that "knows every hair on my head and every prayer upon my lips before I utter the words." As I gained confidence through this practice, I was able to let go of some of the tension caused by internalizing stress and constantly feeling out of my element. I was beginning to perceive the background order, even in times of chaos and profound transformation when it felt like the world was crumbling under my feet. Astrology is a practice that never ends and always holds elements of surprise.

Eventually I drifted away from Catholicism, and gravitated toward study that was more open to questions concerning the cosmos and the afterlife. This break, and what began my avid interest in energy therapies, is what eventually led me to Chinese medicine. Through my brief association as a student of Chinese medicine, I learned about Acutonics, a methodology that uses the power of vibrational (planetary) sound in conjunction with the energy systems of the body to facilitate health and healing.

Until that time, I had navigated intense upheaval, enduring constant disappointment and feelings of failure in both my personal and professional life. I wanted to integrate my past, the academic degree I had attained in music, with my ongoing passion for astrology and my newfound infatuation with Chinese medicine. To say that finding Acutonics was a "godsend" would be an understatement. Not only did it combine music with the system of Chinese medicine, the music was that of the celestial harmonies in (and beyond) our solar system: Pythagoras's music of the spheres. By all accounts, it is difficult to consider this "coincidence" as anything short of a miracle.

Over the course of time, culminating with *this* work, I have continued to straddle two worlds: living in an environment that fears astrology, or looks down upon it as something devilish, juxtaposed against a community whose developments pioneer the work of medical astrology in a brand new—albeit ancient—form. My life has provided me with the opportunity to bridge and mend two very disparate points of view with the intention of reconciling what shows up as opposition.

No matter what your current stance may be with regard to religious, scientific, political, economic, or ecological views, the message intended by this book is one of healing—and hope. It reminds us that everything exists in relationship to the whole. However far apart our differences may be, we all come from unity, and to unity we are returning.

My current experience is teaching me that the fastest way to facilitate healing in another is by healing yourself (according to the nonlocal elements of reciprocity discussed later in the book). For those already healthy and happy, embrace your good fortune, radiate it, live it to the fullest, and be grateful. If you can find a way to pay your gratitude forward, you will never be disappointed with the return on your investment. For those who feel broken by loss or steeped in "the dark night of the soul," my hope for you is that as you read these pages you will discover the potency for magic and miracles that awaits you on the other side of your pain.

Every bit of challenge, struggle, frustration, delay, disappointment, and deep grief that I have experienced has contributed to my development, and none of it would have made sense if I hadn't been able to view my life through a larger lens and the higher octaves of the soul. The most efficient way I have found to do this is by acknowledging the ongoing rhythm, cycles, and harmonic order inherent in our universe and interpreted for us by astrology.

While astronomy is the language of the cosmos, astrology is the language of the individual's unique connection to it, to the whole of which we all are part. It has enabled me to view my life as the "alchemist." By embracing the negative experiences and trusting in an infinite plan, heartaches have always evolved into positive experiences. Perhaps that is why this book is coming forth at this time. Now more than ever, it is time to trust in the implicate order rather than fear the chaos and destructive forces.

Our current worldview and every system born from it, including medicine, is operating from the premise that when something challenges what we hold dear, we must attack it. Destroy the disease, the enemy, the adversary before it destroys us. But what if we realize that the chaos is just a messenger reflecting our own brokenness and providing us with an invitation to respond differently? The very definition of insanity is repeating the same behavior while hoping for a different outcome. Perhaps it is time to recognize that our worldview not only needs to change, but that the need has arisen *because it is time for a change.*

The chaos and fear we witness in the world today, as well as our response to it, is the result of faulty foundations upon which our whole history has been formulated, and we have followed that formula to fever pitch. Until we remember who we truly are, we cannot heal on a personal or global level. And we cannot know who we truly are unless, and until, we are willing to let go of who we have become.

INTRODUCTION

AUTHENTIC MEDICINE

Thus, all Philosophy is like a tree, of which Metaphysics is the root, Physics the trunk, and all the other sciences the branches that grow out of this trunk, which are reduced to three principles, namely, Medicine, Mechanics, and Ethics.
RENÉ DESCARTES (1596–1650)

As with many disciplines and their terminologies, the field of medicine is such an age-old field of study that we have forgotten its roots. What constitutes true medicine? Where did it originate? The answers to these questions provide a foundation for a fresh look at an ancient art, and open the dialog for further exploration.

The word *medicine* comes from the Latin root *medicina*, defined as "the art or practice of medicine, remedy, cure, clinic, treatment or dosing." It stems also from the Latin word *medeor*, meaning "to heal." The root *med* (or *mad*) can be found in many languages. In middle Persia *madha* means "medical science and wisdom." In Sanskrit, *medha* means "intelligence and wisdom." The ancient Greek word *medos* means "advice," and *medomai*, "to think about."

We also have words such as *meditate*, from the Latin *meditari*, which translates to "rehearse, or to say to oneself." These definitions suggest that continual counsel, discovery, and exploration constitute the original meanings of the word we use today as *medicine*.

Another term we readily associate with medicine is *doctor* or *physician.* In Latin, *docere* means "to lead or to teach," and connects to other words such as *docile,* "one who is easily led or taught," as well as *doctrine* and *indoctrination.* *Physician* comes from the Greek word *physike,* which means "knowledge of nature." The word *physician* refers to one who is skilled in the knowledge of nature (distinct from *technology* or *technique,* from the Greek word *tekne*).

And what of *nature*? Its Latin root is *nat,* and means "to be born," as in the words *natal* and *nativity.*

Now let's have a look at the word *authentic.* From the Latin *authenticus* and from Greek *authentikos* it means "original," "genuine," "principal." From *authentes* it means "one acting on one's own authority," from *autos* "self" plus *hentes* "doer," "being." Together these root definitions suggest that authentic medicine is about exploring, thinking about, and meditating upon nature for the purpose of healing oneself.

The word *heal* goes back to the Old English (Germanic) word *hal,* meaning to "make whole." Thus the original definitions of *health* and *medicine* have to do with developing intelligence and wisdom of nature regarding the subject of healing (or becoming whole). *Physician* means "one who acquires knowledge of nature," a derivative of *birth.*

These understandings instantaneously give birth to a new (but ancient) definition of medicine. Authentic medicine acquires new life through this endeavor—it is reborn—as a process of one's own developing wisdom regarding his or her individual nature as well as nature writ large.

A good example of this understanding can be found in our ancestors' study of the heavens as a means of acquiring all forms of knowledge, including medicine. We have to return to a time when astronomy was an intrinsic part of every system of knowledge, and recognize that the language of the cosmos, known as astrology, can aid an individual's understanding of their connection to the whole.

Many books have been written on astrology and on herbal medicine, with only a few touching upon the correspondences between them. This book is inspired by the Hermetic principle "As above, so below," "As within, so without," as well as Hippocrates' quote: "A physician without a knowledge of the cosmos should not call himself a physician. There is one common flow, one common breathing. All things are in sympathy."

The Science of Planetary Signatures in Medicine rekindles the ancient memory lying dormant in the human body/mind/soul: the ultimate remedy for all disease, illness, and disharmony is the *u* (you) in universe. Instead of just "physician, heal thyself," the remedy becomes "physician, know thyself."

All manner of manifestation is influenced by the invisible realm and contains a stellar imprint known as the *doctrine of signatures* by ancient physicians. Many have applied these signatures to plants, fruits, and vegetables and their medicinal effects on the body. However, little attention has been paid to *planetary* effects on health. The natal chart itself reveals a unique planetary signature, with its own geometric and harmonic proportions.

Examining Pythagorean concepts of number expressed through geometry, music, and astronomy allows us to look at the astrological chart as geometry, as music frozen in time. Therefore, music is a most effective means of restoring harmony to dissonant angles and aspects representing "parts of the self." By freeing up those harmonic relationships, the individual engages an awakening process that not only connects neglected parts of the self, it also awakens one's perception of the greater whole.

This awakening of the self provides access to the intrinsic communication network already existing between humans, animals, plants, earth, and the cosmos. The natural science upon which the ancients drew to advance all manner of living is available to us today. There is much to rediscover, and it requires not only asking the right questions, but questioning what we are certain we already know. Embracing the mystery is the first step toward creating a more wholesome future of medicine.

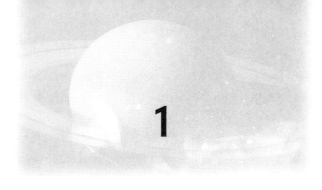

1

ANCIENT COSMOLOGY

To the ancients, studying celestial movement was fundamental to understanding all things related to earthly living. The ordered motion of the stars provided the means for measuring cycles of time and seasons on Earth. But with regard to both time and content, the history we have been taught to accept as humankind's origin is incomplete at best, inaccurate at worst. Archaeological research continues to uncover relics and hieroglyphics that point to a much older history than the one believed to have originated in Mesopotamia (Greek for the "land between two rivers" of the Tigris and Euphrates) around 4000 BCE.

In terms of content, several "splits" or schisms have contributed to incomplete perspectives about our history and human nature. For instance, the splits between astronomy and astrology; chemistry (science) and alchemy (spirit); Eastern history and Western history; and masculine and feminine perspectives all perpetuate half-truths about our multidimensional nature as human beings.

ANCIENT CARTOGRAPHY

For hundreds of years, the Hereford map (circa 1285) perpetuated a half-a-globe representation of the world. This map divides the world into three parts—Asia, Europe, and Africa. Roman Catholicism embraced the Hebrew accounts of Noah's sons (Ham, Shem, and Japheth) being granted these regions. America was not included and there was no mention of a son being granted America. When the Americas were "discovered" by Columbus and put on the map, the church faced an enormous problem.

As scholars wondered how to handle and integrate this new information, a Catholic friar, Jose de Acosta, circulated a story in 1590. He perpetuated "the idea that Siberian hunters crossed an ice bridge upon the Bering Straits to an almost virgin territory bereft of humans and culture."[1] As we will see, a more likely scenario is that humans traveled across the land bridge before sea levels rose, making America one of the oldest continents to exist.

Biblical scholar and theologian Joseph Farrell connects the "Columbus conundrum" to another cover story involving the Fourth Crusade against Constantinople and the Cathars (1204), asserting that Columbus was himself a Templar.[2] The French Templars had formed an alliance with the Republic of Venice around 1200, and it was the Templars' mission to secure Constantinople for its wealth. The Templars wanted to secure hidden cartographic knowledge, "a possibility which is increased by the fact that the post-Fourth Crusade Venetian *podesta* was a member of the Zeno family, which subsequently undertook the voyages to the New World with Prince Henry Sinclair."[3]

According to this account, Columbus's story "to find 'a shorter route to the spice islands'" was itself a cover story because he had visited the Americas several times prior to 1492. Also interesting is an assertion that Ruggero Marino makes about Marco Polo's voyages to the Orient between 1271–1295, which were politically, religiously, and financially subsidized in similar fashion to that of Columbus's expedition.[4] Polo had close ties to both the Templars and the papacy, but was later imprisoned over a conflict between Venice and Genoa in 1296. While he was incarcerated, the first edition of his book was suppressed because, Farrell asserts, it describes an island that was understood to be Japan, but in reality was too far away from China to have been Japan. Polo's description of the natives also paralleled that of Columbus's description of the people he later found in America.[5] Presuming this account to be true, it is likely that Polo had written about America rather than "Cipango," and both the Church and Templars became aware of the existence of the Americas as of 1295. However, if made public knowledge before the "appointed time," this revelation would have threatened the Church's authority.[6]

TEMPLAR SECRET BLOOD AND TREASURE

Farrell also presents a curious hypothesis regarding discrepancies between the Templars' public "mission statement," which was to protect pilgrims traveling to the Holy Land, and a more secret mission having to do with protecting information about their bloodline and ties to a secret Order of Initiates trained in alchemy. The Templars were reputed to have great wealth in their possession, which some believe may have come from the Temple of Solomon, secret excavations under the Temple Mount, or the secrets of alchemy itself. King Solomon's Temple was the first Jewish temple in Jerusalem (circa1000 BCE). About four hundred years later, after the Babylonian king Nebuchadnezzar destroyed it and sent the Jews into exile, Temple Mount was built in what is now the Old City Jerusalem. Whatever historical evidence or secret treasure may be buried there, excavation is strictly forbidden by the Islamic council which now oversees the territory.[7]

During the thirteenth and fourteenth centuries any knowledge regarding a secret bloodline or alchemy would have annihilated the Order of Initiates because it would have opposed church doctrine. Ironically, that is what ultimately did happen, and the highest initiates were gruesomely tortured and put to death around 1310. Addressing this subject in *The Secret Teachings of All Ages,* mystic and researcher of ancient traditions Manly P. Hall (1901–1990) explains that it was the Templars' knowledge about Christianity's early history that caused their persecution and final demise.[8] And what might that knowledge be? Information about discrepancies of the birth, life, and death of Jesus.

One of the accounts relating to these discrepancies is given to us by St. Irenaeus, who was bishop of Lyons in approximately 180. In *Against Heresies,* St. Irenaeus makes the declaration "on the authority of the Apostles," that Jesus lived to teach into his elder years, and was not, in fact, crucified.[9] Another account, published by Bernard H. Springett, a Masonic author, in *Secret Sects of Syria and the Lebanon,* describes how

Jehovah favored the propagation and prosperity of the Essenes. They were visited by a chief of the angels, who commanded in the voice of God that an heir be produced. After four generations Joseph and Mara gave birth to Joshua in Nazareth; he reestablished the ancient religion and restored forgotten religious practices.[10]

Mark Amaru Pinkham, researcher and author of *Return of the Serpents of Wisdom,* states that Jesus was indoctrinated in, and later became the highest priest of the Essene Order. According to Pinkham, he was anointed "Priest King of the Earth" after an Egyptian rite of passage during which he experienced a symbolic death and resurrection. The initiation, which lasted for three days, resulted in his achieving the highest state of consciousness ever conferred upon any mortal being; however, it did not involve any kind of crucifixion.

Hall described another account by Justin Martyr, written in the "First Apology" (circa the second century CE), in which the Crucifixion was addressed as a parallel between the account of Jesus's life in the Christian scriptures and the many saviour-gods of the preceding pagan era.[11] Hall suggested that "First Apology" was written in such a way to make the conversion of Greeks and Romans to Christianity an easier transition. With regard to Christ's "Immaculate Conception" and "Ascension" Martyr explained that it was no different from pre-Christian beliefs about Mercury being the celestial messenger of God (known as Hermes to the ancient Greeks). In addressing pagan objections to Christ's Crucifixion, Martyr explained that it was similar to what they believed had happened to the sons and deities of Jupiter (known as Zeus to the ancient Greeks).

In another publication titled *Seven Books of History Against the Pagans,* circa 418, Christian theologian Paulus Orosius had rendered another version, at the direction of St. Augustine (Bishop of Hippo in North Africa), describing "a divinely ordained movement of imperial power and inspired knowledge . . . gradually from east to west. Adam and Eve's banishment from the terrestrial paradise at the earth's Oriental extreme was the original movement in a series of events that brought human civilization—via India, Babylon, Persia, and Greece—to its ultimate geographical and moral end in Christian Rome."[12]

These different iterations of history contributed to European's confidence in claiming that the Americas were as yet uncivilized, and in need of education and culture. They are partially responsible for the justification of much of the degradation and violation of indigenous populations throughout North and South America. The real history of the American continents is far more ancient than originally believed. We find remnants of that history through the astronomical and cosmological records of the native peoples, which will be further discussed later in this book.

ANTIQUITY OF HUMANITY

Records exist that depict Earth's movement through the precession of the vernal equinoxes, moving at a rate of 30 degrees in 2,160 years. In the opposite direction, west to east, taking 25,920 years, is the cycle of the Milky Way galaxy. This great cycle, as well as the cosmic year, was observed and recorded by indigenous populations from every corner of the globe, including the Americas. For example, the Mexico-Maya of Central America and southern Mexico measured cycles that were literally "astronomical," up to 10, 240,000,000,000 tuns (a 360-day year). Their system is so unique, complex, and accurate, that it confounds modern astronomers. It also clearly demonstrates that the American continents were inhabited for hundreds of thousands of years before recorded history would have us believe.

TABLE 1.1. LENGTH OF TIME ASSOCIATED WITH CYCLES

Cycle	Length of Time
Galactic (or Cosmic) Year	225–250 million years
Precession of the Zodiac Ages	25,920 years
Each Age of the Zodiac	2160 years
Annular Cycle (Yearly)	365 days
Lunar Cycle (Monthly)	28–30 days
Diurnal Cycle (Daily)	24 hours

Source: From Dietrich, *The Culture of Astronomy.*

In fact, author and Greek Classics historian Thomas K. Dietrich states that the "new world" is the "old world." Long before Europeans visited American soil, there are records of Chinese and Japanese vessels having visited the Pacific Rim. In Kennewick, Washington, the remains of a ten- to twenty-thousand-year-old man were discovered. Upon examination, the skeletal structure turned out to be from the Jomon period in Japan (approximately 14,500 BCE–300 BCE). Other, much older examples have been discovered.[13]

Pedra Furada, Brazil (1963, 1988): artifacts 50,000 years old

Minnesota Minnie (1932): skeleton 20,000–25,000 years old

Lewisville Man, Texas (1956): approximately 37,000 years old

Tepexan Man/Tlatilco Skulls (Mexico): 10,000–12,000 years old

Monte Verde, Chile: buildings, streets, sidewalks, and relics dating to 31,000 BCE—the oldest agricultural settlement in the world

The reality is that the ancient world was a maritime culture. Indeed, we need only recall the long voyages of the Chinese treasure fleets of the 1420s when the Chinese emperor sent huge fleets around the world, including the Americas, leaving relics on its coasts and at the mouths of major rivers. This history serves as another telling example of the prevalence of sea travel at this time.

In *Maps of the Ancient Sea Kings*, Professor Charles Hapgood published a collection of antique maps by Swedish scholar A. E. Nordenskjold, including depictions of the Americas thousands of years before Columbus "discovered" them.[14] Demonstrating advanced knowledge, these maps used projection techniques that, until the late Renaissance, were unparalleled. (Perhaps these were the same maps that had been sought by the Templars.) Of great significance is that, according to Dietrich, these maps were reputed to be the work of Agathodaemon, third god of Egypt's First Dynasty dating back 36,525 years.[15] There is clearly more to our history that deserves further scrutiny.

MATRIARCHAL MYTHS,
PATRIARCHAL PERSPECTIVES

We also discover that cultural changes have always coincided with cosmic cycles as the Earth changes its "perspective" from one age to another. To understand these changes, we have to understand the language of the cosmos. As previously pointed out with *medicine,* the word *astrology* has been used in such a way that we have forgotten its connection to our cultural development.

According to Dietrich, ancient people were not "sun worshipers," which implies a more patriarchal association. Rather, they regarded the galaxy as a mother who provides sustenance to the people of Earth. In *The Origin of Culture and Civilization,* Dietrich makes the point that the diurnal cycle was associated with masculine energy given that it concerns itself with daily activity required for survival. The greater cycle was associated with feminine energy as it nurtures (and gives birth to) the shorter and more immediate cycle. The Iroquois of North America are one example of an ancient matriarchal society that has preserved this heritage to the present day. The Cherokee, who possessed advanced knowledge in math and astronomy, claimed an ancestry from the Seven Sisters of the Pleiades. In many of these cultures, as well as in Egypt, Mexico, India, East Asia, and North America, sky goddesses are depicted as feathered serpents and dancing dragons.

In *The Return of the Serpents of Wisdom,* author Mark Pinkham writes about his visit to Machu Picchu, also known as the Temple of the Condor, reminding us that many Incan sites were created in the forms of a condor, snake, or puma. Andean researchers designate the site as an astronomical observatory, while local shamans call it the "crystal city" due to the high concentration of quartz crystal within its granite blocks.[16] Legends connected to this culture suggest that the ninth and most evolved of the priest kings, Pachacutec, revived Machu Picchu with powerful ceremonies and initiations during his reign between 1438 and 1472. An order of priestesses is said to have been established during that time, and reputed to have been endowed with supernatural powers, including the ability to fly.[17]

Although most of recorded history comes to us through the writings of men, ancient societies that seeded Greco-Roman culture recognized the power of the feminine perspective to bring balance and empowerment to an individual's life. Moreover, they recognized that the two perspectives were inextricably entwined in a dance of energy and cosmic cycles, reflected in clockwise and counterclockwise motions simultaneously.[18]

TABLE 1.2. ASTRONOMICAL CYCLES

Rotation	Direction
Diurnal (Daily) Rotation	clockwise (moves backward through zodiac)
Annular (Yearly) Rotation	counterclockwise (moves forward through zodiac)
Vernal Equinox (Precessional)	rotation/clockwise (moves backward through zodiac)
Milky Way Galaxy (MWG)	rotation/counterclockwise (moves forward through zodiac)

Source: From Dietrich, *The Culture of Astronomy*, page 142.

The astronomical account of Adam and Eve shows that many ancient cultures depict a man and a woman side by side in a garden during the Age of Gemini, 6480–4320 BCE. In Egypt, the man and woman were Shu and Tefnut. Eve (the moon and Cancer, the previous zodiac age), was taken from Adam (Gemini, neighbor to Cancer, representing the Tree of Life and home of the serpent of knowledge).[19]

In *Isis Unveiled*, H. P. Blavatsky (1831–1891), co-founder of Theosophical Medicine, explained that the original Hebrew meaning of the word *vah* refers to Adam and Eve: *Jod* ("Yodh") and *Vau* ("He-Va"), "the female serpent as a symbol of Divine Intelligence proceeding from the ONE-Generative or Creative Spirit."[20] (Recall the previous quote from Hall on page 7 regarding Jesus's birth representing an heir to the "voice of Jehovah.") The prophetic "Fall of Man," when understood through an "alchemical" lineage and language, is the separation of woman from man, matter from spirit, and human beings from their Creator.

According to Mark Pinkham in *The Return of the Serpents of Wisdom,* when Jesus returned to Palestine after his training in Egypt, he set about restoring the Essene Order, which had been outlawed by King Herod during his absence. He rallied the twelve apostles, who represented the twelve signs of the zodiac and the twelve phases of soul evolution. When he was grouped with the apostles, totaling thirteen, this number represented the resurrected dragon/phoenix, the number of the planet Venus, and the esoteric number of the androgynous Son of God.

In artistic renditions of the Last Supper, Jesus sat in the center, with six "masculine" astrological signs to his right and six "feminine" astrological signs to his left. In this depiction (for example, by Leonardo da Vinci), Jesus was demonstrating that he had achieved the balanced state of the masculine/feminine union.[21] While spiritual in its context, the medicinal relevance of this information becomes clear when we recall that, as described in the Bible, Jesus personified the ultimate healer. Within the context of his Egyptian training and initiation, he attained that ability through the mastery of the serpent fire.

THE ALCHEMICAL LINK TO MEDICINE

Exploration of ancient astronomy brings with it the realization that science and spirit are twin aspects that can be applied to all systems of knowledge. Astronomy, or planetary nature, is linked to alchemy, which goes to the heart of healing because it addresses the process of change. Alchemy has two expressions: an inner expression (esoteric) and an outer expression (exoteric). These expressions can also be characterized as feminine (inner/hidden/esoteric) and masculine (outer/visible/exoteric). Esoterically, the process of alchemy represents the transformation of a lower to a higher state of human consciousness. Exoterically, the process of alchemy represents the transformation of base metals into gold.

As a society, we have put more emphasis on the exoteric expression insofar as developing "artificial" science to modify natural substances (in hopes of improving upon nature). Even our spiritual development has taken on a certain "prescribed" doctrine that potentially undermines the individual's unique spiritual expression. But the esoteric nature of human beings is as natural as it is ancient. The process of changing our inner state of being naturally changes our external constitution. Alchemy and its formulas were handed down through secret societies and priesthoods by the world's elite, as well as by those entrusted to keep it from being exploited. This circle includes women, who, unfortunately, have been left out of the historic equation for the most part. (Women hierophants and priestesses, in some cases, predated written records.)

The Astor Library of New York (also known as the New York Public Library) has a facsimile of an Egyptian medical treatise that dates back to the sixteenth century BCE. Addressing its authenticity, the nineteenth-century *New-York Tribune* wrote that the papyrus "bears internal evidence of being one of the six Hermetic Books on Medicine, named by Clement of Alexandria."[22] According to the editor of the *Tribune,* Egyptian priests attributed forty-two books to Hermes Thuti (Thoth). Thirty-six of these contained the history of all human knowledge and the last six pertained to anatomy, pathology, surgery, and medicine.[23] As old as this treatise is, the author points out that mankind's history of alchemy, magic, and medicine predates anything any writer can authentically date.

Blavatsky reinforces this connection with alchemy in another example, that of Odin, the Nordic priest and king (circa seventy years BCE), who has historically been credited as the original practitioner of magic in Norse mythology. Yet Nordic mythology shows that he sought guidance from female priestesses called *valas* who "were greatly anterior to his age."[24] Scandinavian archaeology has also uncovered wands and valuable grave offerings that provide evidence that these valas were highly revered by their society.

In ancient Greece, other women rarely written about, such as the female hierophants of Thessaly and Epirus, practiced the "rites of Sabazius." *Sabazios* is identified with *saba* (as in *Sabbath*) and *Zios* (from the Phrygian *dyeus,* precursor to Latin *deus,* the Greek *Zeus,* and

Dionysus). The secrets of these priestesses are still preserved for those who understand the language of nature and soma.[25]

COSMIC LAW

In *The Culture of Astronomy,* Dietrich posits that cosmic law informs natural law.[26] Cosmic law expresses the inherent order, harmony, and interrelationship of all things. The ancients believed that the heavens were the divine expression and means of communication between humans and their Creator. They believed that the human body, created in the image of the cosmic body of the Creator, was imbued with divine characteristics.

Not only the human body but Earth as a celestial body moving through the precession of the equinoxes experiences the attributes of the twelve zodiacal houses that represent the cosmic body: Aries (head), Taurus (neck), Gemini (shoulders/arms), Cancer (breasts), Leo (heart),

TABLE 1.3. PRECESSION OF ZODIAC AGES

Precession of the Zodiac Ages	Associated Symbol	Part of Body
Capricorn 21,600–19,440 BCE	Goat	Knees
Sagittarius 19,440–17,280 BCE	Archer/Centaur	Hips/Thighs
Scorpio 17,280–15,120 BCE	Scorpion	Genitals
Libra 15,120–12,960 BCE	Scales	Lumbar
Virgo 12,960–10,800 BCE	Virgin	Intestines
Leo 10,800–8640 BCE	Lion	Heart
Cancer 8640–6480 BCE	Crab	Breasts
Gemini 6480–4320 BCE	Twins	Shoulders/Arms
Taurus 4320–2160 BCE	Bull	Neck
Aries 2160 BCE–0	Ram	Head
Pisces 0–2160 CE	Fishes	Feet
Aquarius 2161–4320 CE	Man with pitcher of water	Ankles

Source: Derived from Dietrich, *The Origin of Culture,* page 200.

Virgo (intestines), Libra (forearms, navel, lumbar), Scorpio (genitals, reproductive system), Sagittarius (thighs), Capricorn (knees), Aquarius (calves, ankles), and Pisces (feet).[27]

Examining this part of history, storytelling and myths were used as a means of handing down secret knowledge throughout the generations so that it could be revealed to the elect and concealed from those who were not aligned with its teachings. One of these myth writers, Nonnos, was born in Egypt (after Pharaonic Egypt had come under the influence of the Hellenistic period of Greece under Alexander and then the Roman Empire during the Ptolmeic-Roman period) and lived around 500 CE. As an Alexandrian poet, his culture influenced him to write about the ancient knowledge to which he had been indoctrinated, which resulted in the publication *Dionysiaca*.[28] "The Dionysiaca effectually reveals a way of looking at things that only a few of the most select people are ever allowed to see. Just as the era of dark antiquity was shutting its doors, Nonnos brought forth the hierophant's dream, a display of sacred knowledge only discussed within the circle of the exalted cosmologers of the Inner Temple. His work became the tell-all novel of antiquity that binds together religion, history, myth, astronomy, science, and culture into one revealing tableau."[29]

Not to be taken literally, the following description connects the birth of the first god, Dionysus, with the age of Sagittarius (cosmic thigh), and the birth of Athena with that of Aries (cosmic head): According to Dietrich's calculations in *The Origin of Culture,* the Age of Sagittarius would have occurred between 19,440–17,280 BCE.[30] Each age (constellation) lasts 2,160 years and (as articulated in table 1.3), we will be entering the Age of Aquarius around 2160. "Cut the incision in his thigh, and carried him in his man's womb . . . and well he remembered another birth, when his own head conceived, when his temple was big with child . . . until he shot out Athena scintillating in her armor."[31]

Since the ancients corresponded the human body with the cosmic body, the methods of mythology were expressed with phrases such as "the head of the cosmic body," referring to the sign of Aries. These astro-mythological accounts provide invaluable information about our ancient past, which would otherwise be lost. Ancient cosmologers, guided by the precessional clock, used descriptions that corresponded with that particular zodiac sign and era, providing important clues that scientists can now link to historic events.[32]

In the following example, Nonnos describes a time that cataclysmic changes on the Earth occurred "when Leo and Cancer occupied different positions in the heavens. Personified as a battle between Zeus and Typhon, the 'mantle of the earth' was destroyed and the stars and constellations shifted from their 'accustomed positions in the heavens.'"[33]

> Then Nature, who governs the universe and recreates its substance, closed up the gaping rents in earth's broken surface, and sealed once more with the bond of indivisible joinery those island cliffs which had been rent from their beds. No longer was there turmoil among the stars. For Helios replaced the maned Lion, who had moved out of the path of the zodiac . . . Selene took the Crab [Cancer], now crawling over the forehead of the heavenly Lion, and drew him back opposite cold Capricorn, and fixed him there.[34]

In another account, he describes the changing constellations:

> The many [serpentlike] hands of Typhon . . . throttled Cynosuria [constellation] . . . one gripped the . . . Bear's mane as she rested on heaven's axis . . . another caught the Oxdrover [constellation] and knocked him out; another dragged Phosphoros [Venus], and in vain under the circling turning-post [the Sun] . . . held the Bull [Taurus] . . . with a long arm he grasped . . . Aigoceros [Capricorn] . . . he dragged the two fishes [Pisces] out of the sky . . . he buffered the Ram [Aires] . . . [35]

While Western history and science now relegates these tales to the fanciful, there are those whose research suggests the actual existence of certain mythical figures and places. The Apocrypha, disputed as the final part of the Bible, also makes reference to many of these same symbolic representations. And apocryphal texts, which actually imply matters that are secret, occult, or hidden rather than dealing with issues of annihilation (as they are commonly interpreted), offer us a new revelation about our past and our future. (Breaking down the word *apocryphal*, we have *apo* and *cryphal*, the latter *cryphal* being from the feminine of *kryptos*, meaning "hidden.")

THE MYTHICAL LAND OF MU

Ancient remains of an agricultural Chilean city date back to approximately 31,000 BCE. It shouldn't come as a surprise that there might have existed ancient "lost" civilizations, two of which are known as Lemuria (Mu) and Atlantis. Colonel James Churchward (1851–1936) spent fifty years deciphering Naacal tablets he had found in India, with the aid of a friend who knew the Naga-Maya language. Despite the dismissal of his Lemurian hypothesis by modern science, the story provides a fascinating parallel to the Creation story found in the Bible. The first tablet begins with these words: "Originally, the universe was only a soul or spirit. Everything was without life—calm, silent, soundless. Void and dark was the immensity of space. Only the Supreme Spirit, the great Self-existing Power, the Creator, the Seven-headed Serpent, moved within the abyss of darkness. The desire came to Him to create worlds and He created worlds; and the desire came to Him to create the earth, with living things upon it, and He created the earth and all therein."[36]

The seven-headed serpent, as the text further explained, had seven superlative intellectual commands. Stories featuring serpents are represented in every indigenous culture, including those of Egypt and China. The Bible features serpents also. (The word *naga* from the Naga-Maya language translates as "serpent.")

Taking into account that ancient civilizations viewed the heavens as the cosmic body of the Creator, it seems that the "seven-headed serpent" can be referred to the seven "original planets" in our solar system (five planets plus the two luminaries, the sun and the moon). The "serpent" was simply their way of describing the coiled, spiraling motion of the heavens. Remember, too, that the ancient races saw the Milky Way as matriarchal, and used the symbols of serpents and dragons to depict this feminine attribute. The whole—represented by the serpent-like spiral—contained within it (gave birth to) what Blavatsky described as "Seven Sons." They were also called the "Seven Sublime Lords" and "Seven Creative Spirits" that in Hebrew are called the *Elohim,* and who are responsible for the creation of our solar system.[37]

In *The Cosmic Serpent,* anthropologist Jeremy Narby states that the winged serpent found in ancient symbology is sometimes depicted as a dragon. He continues to explain that the dragon, according to *Dictionary of Symbols,* means "the union of two opposed principles."[38] Narby says that a flying serpent represents a paradox, as in the Aztec name Quetzalcoatl: *coatl* means both "serpent" and "twin." Narby can be seen as making reference to not only the dual nature of the primordial Creator but the double helix in human DNA as well as kundalini energy, also known as serpent fire. It is precisely this kind of energy that can be linked to alchemy and the sacred rites of the priests and priestesses of the ancient past.

ALCHEMICAL TRANSFORMATION

Pinkham reiterates for us that alchemy is defined by both the exoteric process of turning base metals into gold, and the esoteric manifestation of the serpent fire that can turn humans into gods and goddesses. When describing Jesus's Egyptian rite of passage, or initiation (mentioned previously), he makes the same connection between serpent fire energy and *kundalini.*

> . . . Jesus was escorted through the paws of the Sphinx and into the Holy of Holies . . . he was directed by the presiding Djedhi to lay down within the ancient sarcophagus while the mantras of Thoth-Hermes were recited over the "corpse." The fiery transformational process of the upward Kundalini was then officially consummated. When Jesus finally arose from his "tomb" three days later he did so as a resurrected Djedhi . . . Having succeeded in achieving a level of consciousness higher than any other soul on Earth, Jesus was anointed not only a Djedhi priest but Grandmaster over the entire Worldwide Order of Serpents . . . He had become a Christ, which with its hard K sound designated Jesus an immortal Serpent of Wisdom.[39]

Through the process originally handed down by Thoth-Hermes, European alchemists learned to make this "serpent fire" in both powder and liquid forms, with the latter being called the elixir of immortality.[40] Both processes involved the use of planetary metals and refers to the idea of a super astronomy that not only heals, but reverses the aging process.

ALCHEMICAL SYMBOLOGY

The serpent symbol described earlier is not found only in astro-mythological history. In medicine and chemistry we have the symbol of the serpent as well. In medicine, we have the Rod of Asclepius and the caduceus, from the Rod of Hermes/Thoth (see figs. 2.2 and 2.3 on page 80). In chemistry, the serpent eating its tail is also represented by the benzene ring. The nineteenth-century chemist Kekule repeatedly dreamed of a serpent eating its tail and discovered the structure of the chemical benzene, which is a ring of six carbon molecules attached to each other, each with four covalent bonds. The benzene ring, also called ouroboros (see fig. 1.1), is the fundamental chemical unit of which complex biochemicals are made. These biochemicals include all the chemical building blocks that make life possible.

In *The Philosophers' Stone*, Joseph Farrell writes about the astrological

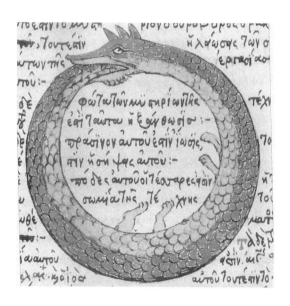

Fig. 1.1. Ouroboros. Drawing by an anonymous medieval illuminator, from a late medieval Byzantine Greek alchemical manuscript.

link to alchemy, showing that the "operations" are described by sign symbols, and the metals are linked to the planets.[41]

TABLE 1.4. ALCHEMICAL ASSOCIATIONS

Operation	Symbol	Zodiac Sign
Calcination		Aries, the Ram
Congelation		Taurus, the Bull
Fixation		Gemini, the Twins
Solution		Cancer, the Crab
Digestion		Leo, the Lion
Distillation		Virgo, the Virgin
Sublimation		Libra, the Scales
Separation		Scorpio, the Scorpion
Ceration		Sagittarius, the Archer
Fermentation		Capricorn, the Goat
Multiplication		Aquarius, the Water-Carrier
Projection		Pisces, the Fishes
Base Metal	**Symbol**	**Planet**
Gold	☉	Sun
Silver	☽	Moon
Copper	♀	Venus
Iron	♂	Mars
Mercury	☿	Mercury
Lead	♄	Saturn
Tin	♃	Jupiter

Source: Farrell, *Philosopher's Stone*, pages 33–34.

What is helpful, if not required, is having a language that provides a road map for understanding the human being's connection to the cosmos. This language is the relevance astrology brings to the process of responding to the larger cycles and hierarchical influence. It also facilitates understanding in the application of the doctrine of signatures to each human's life and, as applied by both Paracelsus and physician and polymath Agrippa Von Nettesheim (aka Henry Cornelius Agrippa, 1486–1535), provides alchemical information about the process of healing.

Despite its controversy, we have to consider the longevity that has been demonstrated by astrology. While its popularity has waxed and waned over the centuries, like the moon, it remains ever present, orbiting the mainstream.[42] For this reason alone it deserves consideration as part of the historical, medical, and philosophical milieu of human inquiry.

THE THREEFOLD NATURE OF HOROSCOPES AND HUMANS

In her book *The Influence of the Zodiac Upon Human Life,* Eleanor Kirk (1831–1908) reminded us that the human constitution is threefold in nature: spirit, soul, body (or father, mother, son), and echoes the Hermetic terms *objective, subjective,* and *passive.*[43] Within the context of astrology, these attributes were expressed amongst the three zodiac signs that are assigned to each of the four elements:

> **Fire** – Aries, Leo, Sagittarius
> **Earth** – Taurus, Virgo, Capricorn
> **Air** – Gemini, Libra, Aquarius
> **Water** – Cancer, Scorpio, Pisces

Regarding spirit, soul, and body, Kirk states that the mind has power over matter: " . . . there is a mind more interior than the animal mind . . . quickened by the solar fluids or planetary action, for it is the genius of the natural man. And there is a still more interior mind, the spiritual, which is absolute over all earthly or planetary conditions, which glows and continues to ripen the divine human into celestial man . . . The stars may influence us, but God rules the stars, and when man recognizes God in himself, he can be dominated no longer by anything apart from God."[44]

Kirk's book addresses relationships between people of different elements, stating that those who are not practiced in the art of evolving and transcending certain weaknesses should carefully choose mates according to harmonious resonance. Although she does not address health per se, her work is relevant for two very important reasons. Elements and their modes (modes meaning the same here as "triune" nature) contribute to the resonance or dissonance (among other combinations of elements/modes), and applies to the body constitution as well as external relationships; and it is always incumbent upon the individual to work with their elemental nature for the purpose of spiritual maturation and physical health.

Also important is that no one element or single event holds the answer for the state of disease or restoration. Neither can we say that there is only one medical system or "magic bullet" that will provide relief. It is always a combination of factors that culminate to reach a point of extreme (*crescendo* to use an Italian term in musical notation) as well as the return to *cadence* ("harmonic resolution") and health. Without practice, there remains an inability to recognize warning signs (symptoms in body or mind) that help one tune into the body as an instrument built for change. In the following passage, Agrippa offers this description of the elements in relationship: "So the earth agrees with cold water, the water with moist air, the air with fire, the fire with the heaven in water; neither is fire mixed with water, but by air; nor the air with the earth, but by water. So neither is the soul united to the body, but by the spirit; nor the understanding to the spirit, but by the soul. So we see that when Nature hath framed the body of an infant, by this very preparative she presently fetcheth its spirit from the Universe."[45]

This description gives the process through which, at the time a person is born, the body is imbued with the four elements while the soul/spirit is brought forth from the universe. Not only does astrology provide a language illustrating the human to cosmos connection, it provides information that links stellar influences upon the natural medicine provided by Earth's plants, minerals, and crystals.

PLANETS, PLANTS, AND PRECIOUS STONES

Sixteenth century Christian mystic and theologian Jacob Boehme (1575–1624) wrote that everything in the manifested world contains within it properties of the seven originally known planets in our solar system. He referred to seven forms in nature, which hold both an eternal and external nature, stating that it is from the eternal that all things external proceed. "The ancient philosophers have given names to the seven planets according to the seven forms of nature; but they have understood thereby another thing; not only the seven stars, but the sevenfold properties in the generation of all essences. There is not anything in the Being of all beings, but it has the seven properties in it, for they are the wheel of the centre . . . The seven forms are . . . Saturn . . . Jupiter . . . Mars . . . Sol . . . Venus . . . Mercury . . . Luna . . . "[46]

In Agrippa's *Occult Philosophy: Natural Magic*, Agrippa explained how the doctrine that proceeds from the heavenly bodies is not one-way only. While humans, plants, and animals receive a stellar imprint that interacts with life on Earth, life on Earth also reverberates into the higher octaves, emphasizing the reciprocity that exists between all life-forms.

All Stars have their peculiar natures, properties, and conditions, the Seals and characters whereof they produce, through their rays . . . in elements, in stones, in plants, in animals, and their members; whence every natural thing receives, from a harmonious disposition . . . some particular Seal, or character, stamped upon it . . . Every thing, therefore, hath its character pressed upon it by its star for some particular effect . . . these Characters contain and retain in them the peculiar Natures, Virtues, and Roots of their Stars, and produce the like operations upon other things . . . and help the influences of their Stars, whether they be Planets, or fixed Stars, or Figures, or celestial Signs . . . "[47]

He referred to terms such as *mutual correspondences* and *sympathies,* referring to language the Greek philosophers used to describe reciprocity: "Now, such kind of attractions, by the mutual correspondency of things amongst themselves, of superiors with inferiors, the Grecians called sympathies . . . you see how by some . . . preparations we are in a capacity to receive certain celestial gifts from above. For stones and metals have a correspondence with herbs, herbs with animals, animals with the heavens, the heavens with Intelligences, and they with divine properties and attributes and with God himself, after whose image and likeness all things are created."[48]

Agrippa's book details the many correspondences among celestial bodies and earthly matter, and a few will be mentioned here. He explains that every plant, stone, or animal is governed by not just one star, but receives influences from many.[49] Tables 1.5 through 1.9 list Agrippa's associations among the plants, herbs, and stones, and their respective planet(s), zodiac sign, and/or star.[50]

TABLE 1.5. ZODIAC SIGNS AND HERBS

Zodiac Sign	Herb
Aries	sage
Taurus	vervaine (verbena) that grows tall
Gemini	vervaine (verbena) that grows bending
Cancer	comfrey
Leo	sow-bread
Virgo	calamine
Libra	mug-wort
Scorpio	scorpion-grass
Sagittarius	pimpernel
Capricorn	dock
Aquarius	dragon's-wort
Pisces	hart-wort

Source for tables 1.5–1.9: Agrippa, *Agrippa's Occult Philosophy,* pages 107–109.

TABLE 1.6. PLANETS AND HERBS

Planet	Herb
Saturn	sengreen
Jupiter	agrimony
Mars	sulphur-wort
Sun	marigold
Venus	wound-wort
Mercury	mullein
Moon	peony

TABLE 1.7. HERMETIC ASSOCIATION OF PLANETS AND HERBS

Planet	Herb
Saturn	daffodil
Jupiter	henbane
Mars	rib-wort
Sun	knot-grass
Venus	vervaine (verbena)
Mercury	cinque-foil
Moon	goose-foot

TABLE 1.8. HERBS WITH PLANETS, SIGNS, OR STAR

Herb	Planet/Sign/Star
Herb dragon	Saturn and Celestial Dragon
Mastic	Jupiter, Sun, Leo
Mint	Jupiter, Sun, Goat Star
Hellebore	Mars, Head of Algol
Moss and sanders	Sun, Venus
Coriander	Venus, Saturn

TABLE 1.9. STONES (GEMS) AND PLANETS, SIGNS, OR STAR

Stone	Planet/Sign/Star
Chalcedon	Mercury, Scorpio, and Capricorn
Sapphire	Jupiter, Sun, and Moon
Emerald	Jupiter, Venus, Mercury, and the star Spica
Amethyst	Mars, Jupiter, and the star Alchamech
Chrysolite	Sun, Venus, Mercury, and the star Falling Vultur
Topaz	Sun, and the star Elpheia
Diamond	Mars, and the head of Algol (star)

It is beyond the scope of this book to enumerate the full variety of all such associations that exist. Instead the reader is directed to seek further knowledge through the resources and references on this subject provided in the bibliography. Specific to herbal medicine without planetary associations, I recommend Hildegard of Bingen's work, mentioned in the next chapter, as a wonderful place to start. For those who are more interested in the planetary associations, the works of Paracelsus and Cornelius Agrippa are excellent resources.

Living in the world without insight into the hidden laws of nature is like not knowing the language of the country in which one was born.

HAZRAT INAYAT KHAN (1882–1927),
SUFI MUSICIAN AND WRITER

2

HISTORY OF HERMETIC MEDICINE

In early antiquity, Egypt had developed well-established systems on all subjects related to human knowledge, suggesting seamless continuity from even hoarier antiquity. As evidence you will recall our mention in chapter 1 of the multivolume Egyptian medical treatise of the sixteenth century BCE, which contains six Hermetic books on medicine. Although it's outside the range of *this* book to detail the history of all physicians relevant to this topic, there are those whose contributions made it possible to revive Hermetic medicine (or keep it alive) at crucial points in history.

The first of these illustrious individuals we must mention is, of course, Hermes Trismegistus, known as Thoth (in ancient Egypt) and as Enoch in the Bible. Genesis 5:21–24 (ESV) says: "And Enoch walked with God and he was not; for God took him." The Books of Enoch pick up where the Bible left off, describing what Enoch saw during his time with God and witnessing the many kingdoms of heaven, including the operation of the planets and stars. The following excerpt, concerning the zodiac, describes the eighth level: "And Gabriel lifted me up . . . And I saw the eighth heaven, which is called in the Hebrew tongue Muzaloth (Zodiac), the changer of the seasons, of drought, and of wet, and of the twelve constellations of the circle of the firmament, which are above the seventh heaven."[1]

With regard to medicine, Enoch became a scribe, assigned with the task of imparting knowledge, including that of medicine, to human beings on Earth. Blavatsky explains that the term *Enochian* means "inner eye" in Greek, and "initiator" and "instructor" in Hebrew, pointing out that Enoch's experience is essentially the same as that written about other prophets. (The Biblical prophet Elijah was also taken into heaven while still alive, and came back to teach celestial knowledge.)[2]

In *The Hermetica* internationally renown authors Timothy Freke and Peter Gandy explain that Thoth was a revered Egyptian sage who possessed such great wisdom that it transformed him into a god. Like Enoch, he became an ambassador between heaven and earth, relaying divine messages to humanity and recording their earthly deeds. He taught the Egyptians astronomy, architecture, geometry, medicine, and religion, and is credited for being the architect of the pyramids. These authors further explain that the Greeks (who learned of Egyptian theology/history/mythology) identified Thoth with their god Hermes. Like Thoth, Hermes was an ambassador between the gods in heaven and living souls on Earth, as well as those transitioning through the underworld. They added the word *Trismegistus* to his name, which means "thrice great"—greatest king, greatest priest, and greatest scribe.[3]

Although its historical development is not well defined, Hermeticism can still be seen to have had a great influence on the development of Western culture and medicine. For our purposes, we will focus primarily on physicians, although most were also philosophers and initiates of divine alchemy encompassing both the esoteric and the exoteric expressions.

To review, alchemy has both an esoteric expression, referring to the transformation of a mortal human into a god/goddess, and an exoteric expression. Exoterically, alchemy refers to the transformation of base metals into gold. It is important to stress the belief that, in order for any success to be made in the exoteric manifestation of gold, the human must first undergo a successful esoteric transformation. This belief provides one reason many physicians were part of secret priest crafts that had mastered many subjects, not the least of which was medicine.

Exoterically, the four base metals alchemists used to turn into gold are tin, lead, mercury, and silver, which are associated with the planets

Jupiter, Saturn, Mercury, and the moon, respectively (see table 1.4). Gold was represented by the sun, which is a likely reason gods were often symbolized by the sun, such as the Greek Apollo and the Egyptian Horus. As mentioned previously in Mark Pinkham's account, the divinity of Jesus Christ also correlated with the sun, and the twelve apostles with the constellations. This correlation between gods and the sun was also noted among groups who were converted to Catholicism during the Roman Empire; first the Romans (such as the Cult of Mithras), and then Celtic societies within the Roman Empire. The assignation of the date of the birth of Jesus at the time of the winter solstice is taken by some to have signified the return of the sun/god in syncretism with the new theology.

APOLLO AND ASCLEPIUS

The National Library of Medicine (NLM) and the National Institutes of Health (NIH) provide their "official" chronological list of physicians throughout Western history (see page 45). The first one listed is Apollo (the aforementioned "sun god"), circa 700 BCE, described as the "bringer and reliever of plagues" as written about in Homer's *Iliad*. Apollo, who had been given the seven-stringed lyre by Hermes, was also

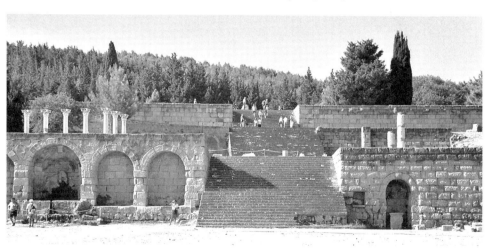

Fig. 2.1. Kos, Asklepeion, Griechenland.
Photograph by Heiko Gorski (CC BY-SA 3.0).

associated with music and known to be the leader of the muses. (The seven strings represent the Elohim, from the Hebrew, and the seven superlative intelligences mentioned earlier.)

Apollo's son, Asclepius, was known in ancient Greece as the god of medicine, and in the *Corpus Hermeticum* is depicted to have learned about the laws of philosophy and medicine from Hermes. The staff of Asclepius, having only one serpent, remains a symbol of medicine today (fig. 2.2); as does the staff of Hermes, which has two serpents; as does the caduceus (fig. 2.3). Once again, the symbol of the snake/serpent is associated

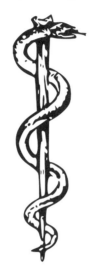

Fig. 2.2. Rod of Asclepius. Art by CatherinMunro, derivative work by Hazmat2 (CC BY-SA 3.0).

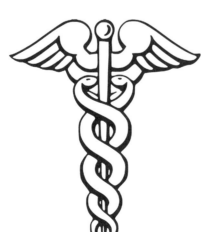

Fig. 2.3. Modern caduceus. By Rama and Eliot Lash.

with medicine. In the case of Apollo and Asclepius, music is associated with medicine as well. This association of music and medicine was durable from the Pythagoreans of ancient Greece to the physicians of medieval Europe.

Asclepius had five daughters, all of whom shared some aspect of the healing work of their father. The first, Hygieia, was the goddess of health, preventer of disease, and personification of cleanliness, whose name became the root for the modern word English *hygiene*. Panacea became the goddess of universal remedy, or "all-heal;" Iasos, the goddess of recuperation from illness; Aceso, the goddess of the healing process; and Aglaea, the goddess of beauty and magnificence. Two of Asclepius's sons, Machaon and Podalirius, became well-known surgeons and medics. Not much is known about his other two sons, Telesphoros, associated with mythology, and Aratus, who is known mainly for a poem he wrote describing celestial phenomenon and the constellations.[4]

PYTHAGORAS

During the sixth century BCE, Pythagoras of Samos lived and had ties to alchemy and Hermetic principles. In *The Music of Pythagoras,* musician and biographical author Kittie Ferguson writes of an interesting connection between Pythagoras and Hermes.[5] Apparently, the Neoplatonist Iamblichus described Pythagoras as a supreme master and witnessed his ability to recall past lives. Pythagoras's first memory was of Hermes' son Aethalides. In this memory, Hermes told his son Aethalides he could choose any gift except that of immortality, and he chose to remember everything that had happened to him in former lifetimes. According to Hall, Pythagoras's own birth was prophesied by the Oracle of Delphi, who described him as one who would surpass all men in beauty and wisdom and contribute much to the illumination of mankind. His disciples called him "The Master," though he called himself a philosopher (lover of wisdom).[6]

Pythagoras's contribution to divine alchemy found its expression in the tetraktys and the four classical elements: earth, air, fire, and water (we will address the fifth element momentarily). To Pythagoras,

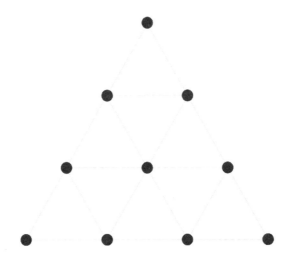

Fig. 2.4. The tetraktys, a mystical, triangular figure important to
the Pythagoreans, consists of ten points arranged in four rows
with one, two, three, and four points in each row.

wisdom was the source of all things, and the height of wisdom was represented by the geometric monad (the highest deity and point on the
tetraktys triangle). From the monad the dyad is produced, and from
the monad and dyad, numbers, points, lines, and two-dimensional and
three-dimensional forms are created.

These lines culminate in the "shapes" or mathematical structures
of the four elements, which form the building blocks for everything in
creation: earth was the cube, air was octahedral, fire was tetrahedral,
and water icosahedral.[7] The fifth element, ether, in the shape of the
dodecahedron, is the twelve-faced symmetrical sphere that represents
the foundation of the universe.[8] Recall, as well, Pinkham's story of Jesus
sitting in the center of the twelve apostles, six to the left and six to the
right, symbolizing the balance of masculine/feminine energies.

Pythagoras regarded the planets as celestial beings, alive and resonating with music/song, and operating according to the divine law
of mathematical order originating in the monad. He believed the
planets were deities, yet subservient to the one first cause.[9] Iamblichus
describes Pythagorean medicine as melodies that soothe the passions

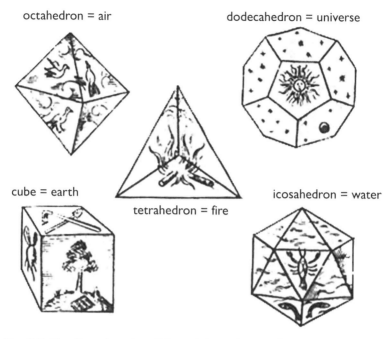

Fig. 2.5. The five platonic solids and their elemental correspondence.

of the soul, including despondency and lamentation.[10] There is a great deal more to consider where Pythagoras is concerned; we will return to him and the subject of math as it relates to geometry, music, astronomy, and medicine a bit later. Briefly mentioned next are those in history whose life work carried on a philosophy of natural science in the West.

THALES OF MILETUS

In 600 BCE, Thales of Melitus, considered one of the Seven Sages in ancient Greece, made contributions to the understanding of nature and physics. He was the first to describe phenomena through nature's processes rather than through metaphor and myths. He believed that all natural matter is imbued with divine life and spirit. More importantly, he believed that water was the divine and creative substance from which all natural matter originated.

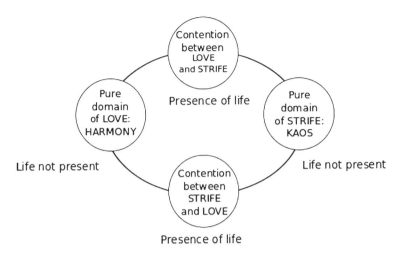

Fig. 2.6. Concept map of "Empedocles' Cosmic Cycle."
Based on the conflict between love and strife.
By Paolo.anghileri (CC BY-SA 3.0).

EMPEDOCLES (490–450 BCE)

Born in 490 BCE, Empedocles became the last pre-Socratic philosopher to record his ideas. His contribution is articulated in the cosmogenic theory of the four elements, proposing that two opposing forces, love and strife, created the mixture and separation of the elements. Like Pythagoras, he believed in reincarnation, describing it as the transmigration of the soul.

Influenced by predecessors such as Pythagoras, he based his work on the simple observation of how the elements tend to manifest in the physical world. Greek philosophy held that life depends upon a combination of all four elements. Earth provides agricultural sustenance and food. Water provides the means by which Earth's plant life grows, allowing it to continue providing sustenance. Without the light of the sun in combination with water, there would be no food, and air and oxygen are required for human life to survive. Having practiced the Hermetic principle, "As above, so below," the Greeks understood that if the elements existed in the external world, they must also exist in human beings.

Although humoral medicine prevailed, and before the separation of science and healing art was completed, Western physicians recognized a primary element called "quintessence" that held all other elements together. Quintessence was understood to be the invisible mover, the life-force energy inherent in all plants, animals, and humans. Once the separation of science and healing took place, quintessence became irrelevant to the practice of medicine.

HIPPOCRATES (460–370 BCE)

In 460 BCE, Hippocrates was born. He is most widely known today for his association with the Hippocratic oath. It begins "I swear by Apollo, the healer, Asclepius, Hygieia, and Panacea, and I take to witness all the gods, all the goddesses, to keep according to my ability and my judgment, the following Oath and agreement . . ."[11] Classic scholar Ludwig Edelstein believed it was actually written by Pythagoreans. Hall writes that while Hippocrates is credited by modern physicians with being the father of medicine, the ancient Therapeutae credits Hermes as the founder of art and healing.

Hippocrates, by all accounts, dissociated medicine from the other ancient sciences of the temple. Specifically, he separated the scientific and spiritual philosophies that remain in effect in Western medicine today. Until that time, they had been part of one system known as Hermetic medicine.

So in that regard, Hippocrates really is the father of modern medicine. He also practiced humoral medicine, which was the science of basing a patient's assessment on the balance of the four elements (also called humors). This practice of humoral medicine predates Hippocrates, with the Greeks owing their development and techniques to Egyptian and Mesopotamian physicians (please refer to *Avicenna's Medicine* for more on this). Humoral medicine was central in Western medicine until the nineteenth century.

In addition to advocating and utilizing humoral medicine, Hippocrates also believed that the human body held within it the power to heal itself.

PLATO AND PHILISTION OF LOCRI

According to British medical historian Vivian Nutton, at the time the *Hippocratic Corpus* was written in the fourth century CE, Plato was formulating his own ideas about medical philosophy. Nutton writes that Plato's writings regarding the explanation of illness ultimately had a lasting impact on Western intellectual minds. While he often mentioned Hippocrates, there was another doctor, Philistion of Locri, to whom he referred in a letter, expressing hopes that this doctor would be allowed by Dionysius II to come to Athens.[12] Nutton explains that, while it's impossible to verify that the two ever met, there were occasions in Plato's travels when he very well could have met the physician.

Nutton also refers to a certain papyrus, the *Anonymous Londinensis,* which alludes to virtual identical medical theories between Plato and Philistion. Nutton describes Philistion's theory of disease as having three causes that could affect the four humors—hot, cold, wet, and dry—and their balance. The first he described as an internal excess or deficiency, the second an external excess or deficiency and/or the presence of wounds or sores. The third cause was described as an obstruction to airflow in or out of the body. If the body did not have enough airflow, decay would ensue; and if the body had too much air, it could cause swelling, excess sweating, or other distress.[13]

GALEN (130–200)

Galen's medicine drew upon such predecessors as Plato, Aristotle, and Hippocrates. He based his medicine upon the four elements and their combinations and contraries—hot, cold, wet, and dry. Influenced by Aristotle's Generation and Corruption, which addresses the question on how things come into being and how they pass away, Galen developed his methods on the material composition of the elements expressed in his work *On Mixtures.*[14]

Plato's influence on Galen produced a physician who accepted the world soul as collective, and the tripartite soul within humans (body/soul/spirit). Today, we use the terms body/mind/soul or body/mind/spirit; however, "mind" defined by Hermetic principles means something more than rational thinking, as in the "mind of God" who creates with ideas.

Galenic medicine is best known for its application of the humoral theory, which aims to maintain or restore the balance of four expressions in the body. This theory is based on an understanding of four fluids—phlegm, blood, black bile, and yellow bile—and how they correspond to three different body parts : the head with phlegm, the heart with blood, the liver with black bile, and the liver's partner the gallbladder with yellow bile.[15] (For the purposes of our discussion the liver and gallbladder are deemed to comprise one unit.) The significance of these three parts of the body are also linked to Plato's tripartite soul: the head with Sophia (wisdom), the heart with emotion and spirit, and the liver with desire.[16] It is through the balancing of these principles that the physician helps the patient to prevent disease and promote wellness.

A DIGRESSION INTO CULTURAL INFLUENCES ON MEDICAL PRACTICES

Before we continue our examination of these seminal figures, it's important to understand some cultural influences on the spread of medical practices throughout the world. From 632–1200, Islam's presence in Egypt, North Africa (into Spain), and the Middle East perpetuated the study of Greek medicine and the translation of Greek texts into Arabic. Islamic culture became instrumental in the transference of ancient Greek medicine and philosophy from the West to the East (and then back again). Avicenna (930–1037), became known in Europe and the Middle East as one of the most significant contributors to the Islamic golden age.[17]

From 1200–1350, there was a brief renewal of Greek medicine among Western scholars when certain texts were recovered during the Crusades. However, during that tumultuous period, when the Eastern Orthodox Church—which had split off from Rome in the fifth century—was expanding, Hermetic principles disappeared into the shadows and became lost to Western culture until the Italian Renaissance (fourteenth to the sixteenth centuries). It was the work of

Paracelsus (1493–1541) whose contributions were chiefly responsible for the revival of Hermetic philosophy during this period.

With regard to the subject of alchemy, it is relevant to mention his significant success regarding the mixing of tinctures, which came from Hermes Trismegistus and the elixir of the philosopher's stone. Referring to this elixir in his treatise on alchemical medicine Paracelsus states, "The life of many . . . has been extended . . . to several centuries, as is most clearly shewn in different histories . . . though it seems scarcely credible to anyone. For its power is so remarkable that it extends the life of the body . . . and keeps it so firmly . . . that it lives on in safety from all infirmities."[18]

Regarding his own success he states: "So, then, the Tincture of the Philosophers is a Universal Medicine, and consumes all diseases, by whatsoever name they are called, just like an invisible fire. The dose is very small, but its effect is most powerful. By means thereof I have cured the leprosy, venereal disease, dropsy . . . cancer . . . and the whole race of internal diseases, more surely than one could believe. Of this fact Germany, France, Italy, Poland, Bohemia, etc., will afford the most ample evidence."[19]

Paracelsus' method proved to be too magical for widespread trust, and that, combined with a cantankerous personality and the cultural changes of his day, once again would lead to the demise of alchemy.

AVICENNA (980–1036)

Avicenna's chief contribution to the lost art of Hermeticism came from the fact that he brought Greek philosophy to Islam. His publication entitled *The Canon of Medicine* presents the Greco-Arabic-Islamic approach, called Unani medicine, and is regarded as one of the most influential medical books to this day. His objective and major focus was to rid medicine of "superstitious" terms, such as *spirit,* and offer more empirical descriptions of the interaction of the four elements (humors), placing emphasis on prevention of disease and preservation of health. His methods are still being used in traditional Unani (Greco-Arabic) and Ayurvedic medicine in India today.[20]

Consistent with Greek philosophy, Unani medicine recognizes the four classical elements as the major components of all living beings. Just as yin and yang divide to become four elements, so do each of the elements manifest into a combination of two expressions: "Earth is cold and dry, water is cold and wet, air is hot and wet, and fire is hot and dry. Red bile (blood/sanguine) is hot and moist; white bile (phlegm) is cold and moist; yellow bile (choleric) is hot and dry; and black bile (melancholic) is cold and dry. Each individual's normal healthy state will be a unique combination of these four humors."[21]

In *Avicenna's Medicine: A New Translation of the 11th-Century Canon with Practical Application for Integrative Health Care,* Abu-Asab et al. explain how Avicenna's medical practice acknowledged the interaction between celestial influences and physical health.

The aggregation of many bright planets in a region or near the sun may increase temperature substantially, especially when the planets are at their zenith or close to it. When far from their zenith heat is reduced. Zenith effect is influenced by its duration, but not the same effect as proximity. Terrestrial effects are due to latitudes, altitudes, presence of mountains and seas (terrain), wind and soil. Latitudes closer to the tropic of Cancer (north) and the tropic of Capricorn (south) are warmer during their summers than are places closer to the equator or away from the two tropics. For this, the heat is more intense at the end of Cancer, beginning of Leo (July 22–23), when the sun is at its maximum declination. When the sun moves down closer from the zenith of Cancer, it is hotter than if it had remained in the same degree of declination. The sun remains at the orbital nodes of the equator during the equinoxes. Countries that are at the tropics are the warmest. Heat at the equator is not as excessive as when the sun is at its zenith at the tropic of Cancer . . . [22]

HILDEGARD OF BINGEN (1098–1179)

As a twelfth-century Christian mystic, composer, artist, healer, and natural scientist, Hildegard of Bingen received no formal education in science or philosophy. Rather, she developed a comprehensive system of natural medicine from her mystic visions alone. With regard to her lack of education, she is quoted from a letter written in 1146 to Bernhard of Clairvaux saying: " . . . I am an uneducated mortal and am in no way learned in things concerning the external world, but taught from within by means of my soul."[23]

Responsible for compiling a trilogy of books, and over three hundred (known) letters, compositions, and songs, her work demonstrates access to an inner wisdom capable of educating more profoundly than traditional education.[24]

Hildegard's medicine was based on the four elements, and thus considered consistent with the humoral medicine of the time. She offers an anthology of herbal remedies applicable to us today. Physicians, scholars, and authors Wighard Strehlow and Gottfried Hertzka write that, for Hildegard, the four elements represented the key to restoring human health, for their compositions and relations are what determine human constitution, just as it does the construction of the world. " . . . [J]ust as the four elements hold the world together, they also form the structure for the human body. Their distribution and function in the whole human being are such that they constantly sustain the person . . . When the elements fulfill their purpose correctly and orderly, so that warmth, dew, and rain come . . . in good measure and at the proper time . . . , and maintain the earth and its fruits in health, and thus bring bountiful harvests and good health, then the world will prosper."[25]

One of the most interesting characteristics regarding Hildegard's remedies is that they reflect knowledge consistent with Ayurveda, Chinese medicine, and modern Western herbalism despite her lack of training in any formal system.[26]

PARACELSUS (1493–1541)

In Paracelsus we find a controversial and revolutionary physician who vehemently opposed the medical practice of his contemporaries. This posture did not win him many friends, but did develop for him a distinctly cantankerous reputation. Swiss physician, botanist, alchemist, astrologer, and social rebel, he was neither well liked by his peers nor bothered by that fact. He was a radical who shook the foundation of what had become, since the separation of science and spirituality, a system intolerant of "superstitious" practices. The irony is, writes Hall, that his success rate for healing difficult cases far surpassed that of his colleagues.[27]

Paracelsus devoted his life to studying the Hermetic philosophy and to reconciling the art of healing with the religious systems of paganism and Christianity.[28] The Renaissance period, during which Paracelsus lived, brought about a brief resurgence of Hermetic philosophy and, by all accounts, Paracelsus reached a level of mastery in alchemy few physicians have attained before or since.

Like Empedocles, Paracelsus was an avid observer of nature. One of his distinct gifts was that of making the world his laboratory. He believed that physicians should search within for spiritual insight, hold reverence for nature, and actively facilitate the contemplation of mystery as it relates to healing. By tuning into nature in this way, one can perceive how the cycles of growth in plants follow the celestial patterns. For example, some petals open according to the phases of the moon, some to the sun's cycle, and others to distant stars.[29]

According to Paracelsus, the Earth is permeated by a mysterious energy that governs the four elements, and is captured by minerals and metals. His observations led him to conclude that plants derive their energies from nature: the outer atmosphere (including that of the celestial bodies) and the Earth beneath. These secrets he discovered while he was working in mines, gaining much from his observations. More importantly, he listened to the stories other miners shared regarding legends and folklore peculiar to their trade.

The miners explained to him that minerals have a life cycle similar to plants and animals. They shared stories of how men seeking gold in a particular region would find none on their first visit. However, returning several years later to that same place, they would find threads of precious metal having "grown" through the ore.

Instead of dismissing these stories, Paracelsus examined them thoroughly. He made it his mission to understand the mysteries of the four elements, believing that each had an existence apart from humans that was not always visible. He believed that each element has its own world and sphere that interpenetrates the spheres of other elements, while still possessing its own qualities.[30] In other words, he ascribed to each element a twofold expression: one that pertains to cause and is invisible, and one that pertains to effect and is visible. He believed that the causal invisible spheres of these elements were subject to scientific scrutiny, but only if humans developed the internal faculties to see beyond the physical, objective realm.

Hall described Paracelsus as one of the few minds (and physicians, save Ficino) to ever attempt the reconciliation of the religious systems of paganism with Christianity. This distinction renders his contribution irreplaceable as we continue our exploration of planetary medicine and its implications for a more authentic medical paradigm.[31]

NICHOLAS CULPEPER
(1616–1654)

Culpeper was an English botanist, herbalist, physician, and astrologer who spent most of his life outdoors cataloging hundreds of medicinal herbs. He is best known today for his important book, *The English Physician*. Learned in Greek and Latin, he was able to study the ancient medical texts. As the son of a clergyman, he maintained a deep faith in the Creator:

> These qualities in man altered by the various influences of the Stars, the Sphere of the one carrying a swifter motion than the sphere of the other, then various must needs be the disposition of man's body . . . the universal cause of the Crisis is the influence of the Heavens: for the Celestial bodies, either by heat, light, motion, or aspects, configuration, or all of them, or some of them, act not only in the four Elements, but Elementary bodies . . . But if bodies of men are elementary, composed of Fire, Aire, Earth, and Water, he must needs participate in one measure or other, of all these Elements . . ."[32]

With the exception of Avicenna and Hippocrates—who were less inclined toward the spiritual and advocated for empirical methods and terminology—these historical figures acknowledged that the relationship between the cosmos and Earth could be discovered through the spiritual arts. In Galen, Empedocles, Hildegard, Paracelsus, and Culpeper, we find those who cultivated rather than discounted the inner wisdom that connects to soul and spirit. This spirit was recognized as being part of the greater world soul, as taught by Plato, and finding expression in the four elements, planetary bodies, and all the plants, stones, and creatures of the Earth.

Hermeticism and humoral medicine both recognize that change is the key to maintaining balance in the body and among the four elements. Just as Earth reveals its seasonal rhythm, providing just the right change at the right time to sustain life on this planet, so too do humans benefit from allowing change that maintains equilibrium among the four humors. Beyond the annual cycle, we have larger cycles that also affect life on our planet.

As a global society, we are in the midst of transitioning from the Age of Pisces to the Age of Aquarius. A paradigm shift is not only inevitable—it is in order. Understanding smaller cycles within the context of greater ones such as this helps us to respond with trust rather than react with fear, as has been our historical bent. The inherent order revealed through nature all around us is our guiding light—there is no need to improve upon this natural science. We only need to support it so that it, in turn, can sustain our ability to not just survive, but actually thrive. The great Greek philosopher Heraclitus (535–475 BCE) famously said, "The only thing that is constant is change"—one of the wisest quotes known to man.

THE RENAISSANCE

With the fall of Eastern Orthodox Constantinople to the Ottoman Empire in 1453, scholars began moving from Constantinople to Italy, taking the Greek texts with them, and renewing the interest in Greek philosophy and medicine known as the Renaissance.

Not long before that, historically speaking, the Spanish Reconquista of Toledo by the Christians from the Moors in Spain had begun the same process of restoring ancient medical knowledge during the thirteenth–fourteenth centuries.[33]

NEOPLATONISTS

Among those important figures also responsible for restoring and perpetuating Hermetic medicine were Neoplatonists Marsilio Ficino (Italy, 1433–1499), Giordano Bruno (Italy, 1540–1600), and Robert Fludd (England, 1574–1637). While each of these figures deserves more attention and distinction, for these purposes it is practical to describe them as Christians who passionately believed in preserving ancient Hermeticism and for making attempts to harmonize an understanding of the planets (through the language of astrology), math, music, religion, and science. For Bruno, unfortunately, this attempt ended tragically, as he was accused of crimes against the Catholic faith and burned at the stake. Before he died Bruno published many works on mnemonics, one of which was *The Art of Memory* in 1582. Ficino was responsible for translating many Greek texts into Latin, including the *Corpus Hermiticum*, and the writings of several Neoplatonists such as Iamblichus, Ploteny, and Porphyry.

Robert Fludd, who graduated in 1605 with an M.B. and M.D., made several failed attempts to enter the College of Physicians in London, which had just been established in 1596. In 1609 he finally succeeded, and became a prominent "Paracelsian." His knowledge and experience encompassed astrology, math, cosmology, Kabbalism, and Rosicrucianism. He also engaged in many debates concerning Hermeticism with Johannes Kepler (1571–1630) (an astronomer who recorded the movements of the stars and planets, and is credited with discovering the laws of planetary motion, two of which were published in 1609, and the third in 1619.)

This brief resurgence in Hermetic medicine during the Renaissance was also short-lived. Western scholars of that time began to vehemently oppose Greek philosophy, divorce medicine from its ancient origins, and develop the separate roots of modern Western medicine. Thus can be seen the beginning of the current medical model of separation we are experiencing today.

There is an historical pattern, mostly in the West, of discounting beliefs and practices from the preceding ages so that a new belief system could be exalted. Some of this discontinuity can be attributed to the fact that recorded history was handed down by scribes, written symbolically, and not shared with the masses. Eastern cultures, however, such as China and India, as well as indigenous cultures around the globe, have been better able to maintain continuity with the past that gives us a point of reference to explore.[34] Scholars have described Chinese medicine as a system of knowledge that "never threw anything away."

Both esoteric (inner/feminine/spiritual) and exoteric (outer/masculine/material) aspects of alchemy must be remembered, respected, and balanced if we are to succeed in the development and practice of authentic medicine. We will return to this subject later in the book, but as we can see in the example of Hildegard of Bingen (1098–1179) above, information unavailable through books and intellectual pursuits may still be ascertained through inner wisdom.

CHRONOLOGY OF ANCIENT PHYSICIANS*

700 BCE   Homer's *Iliad* recounts that Apollo is the bringer and reliever of plagues.

600 BCE   Thales of Miletus, one of the Seven Sages of Greece, initiates inquiries about nature and physics; thus begins the rise of Greek science and philosophy.

580 BCE   Pythagoras of Samos is born; he later founded a mystical school for science and philosophy. (NIH/NLM use the term *cult*.)

480 BCE   Philosopher and physician Empedocles is born.

460 BCE   Hippocrates is born; later begins the *Hippocratic Corpus*.

384 BCE   Philosopher and scientist Aristotle is born.

334–325 BCE   Egypt, the Middle East, and western India are indoctrinated in Greek knowledge when Alexander the Great conquers these regions.

*Based on information from the National Library of Medicine (NLM) and the National Institutes of Health (NIH), www.nlm.nih.gov/hmd/greek/greek_timelline.html.

330 BCE–100 CE	The city of Alexandria, Egypt, becomes a mecca where scholars from many cultures seek knowledge on philosophy, science, religion, and medicine.
146 BCE	Greek civilization begins exchanges with Rome.
50–70 CE	Dioscorides writes *De materia medica* (Original Greek: Περι ὑλης ιατρικης).
129 CE	Noted physician Galen is born; his medicine is based on the four humors.
150 CE	Artemidorus writes *Oneirocritica* (translation: *The Interpretation of Dreams*).
476 CE	Roman Empire begins to fall and Western physicians lose touch with Greek scholars and Eastern texts.
632–1200 CE	Islam takes over Egypt and the Middle East. Arabic medical scholars study the ways of Greek physicians and translate Greek texts into Arabic.
1200–1350 CE	Texts found during the Crusades renew Western scholars' interest in Greek medicine.
1450–1598 CE	Constantinople falls in 1453, and many Byzantine scholars move to Italy, bringing Greek texts with them; Greek medical texts are intensely studied and printed.
1540–1800 CE	Western scholars question Greek medicine and philosophy. Divorcing medicine from its ancient paradigm they begin to develop modern Western medicine.

3

COSMOLOGICAL ROOTS
OF YIN AND YANG

Although there are differences between Eastern and Western method-ologies, we also find striking similarities among ancient semi-mythical legends that seeded these cultures. They have continued to develop through practice and oral and written traditions in the East. In the West, we lost untold resources when the Library of Alexandria was destroyed circa 270–275 during a period of political and religious tur-moil. Irreplaceable written records of our full, true history literally went up in flames and a new manufactured history took its place.

Since that time, world regimes have represented human civiliza-tions and societies as many unrelated cultures with distinct, and often, irreconcilable values—as the saying goes, "As far as the East is from the West." What we are discovering, however, is that a singular parent cos-mology has influenced them all. At the time Jesus is recorded to have lived, the Alexandrian library kept records of all the oral traditions. According to Acharya S, pen name for D. M. Murdock, author of sev-eral books on comparative religion and mythology, the library was part of an information network that spanned Europe and China.[1]

During the transition to Catholicism, written knowledge was not the only memory that was destroyed. Recall the Hereford map (chap-ter 1), misrepresenting world cartography for many generations, delib-erately excluding the Americas. But history and cartography were not all that were subject to revision; even words were given definitions that rendered meaning quite different from the original. One example pertinent to this discussion is the word *myth*. *Mythos* originally referred to accounts and records of different people about their history, but during the Middle Ages was revised by the Roman Catholic Church to mean "imaginative and fanciful tales veering far from any truthfulness."[2]

Many centuries later archaeological research offers evidence that contradicts the history we were taught to believe, as well as the later imposed definition of myth. For instance, Frank Calvet's discovery in 1865, seven years before Hienrich Schliemann arrived on the scene, collapsed the "myth" of Troy recounted in Homer's *Iliad*. He uncovered not just one city but nine underground layers dating back to thirteenth century BCE.[3] If we consider that mythical accounts often contain merit, this opens wide the door to possibilities, not the least of which is that the East and West have more in common than we originally believed. (And considering that Earth is a sphere, East literally does meet West along the equator.) So while the medieval church may have summarily dismissed certain legends as "veering far from any truth," it might be wise to reconsider these accounts, especially as they relate to world history and cultural development, connections, and commonalities.

While deliberate destruction of written records was a major reason for interrupted history in the West, in China centuries passed before ancient knowledge was written down and recorded. Through oral tradition, practice, and the recording of many Chinese "classics" by the Han period two thousand years ago, which often claimed greater antiquity, Chinese cosmology was preserved.[4] Examining the earliest available forms of information, we find similarities among China, Egypt, Sumer, Africa, and accounts in the Bible. Where China's cosmology is concerned, we will focus on the concept of yin and yang, and especially how it has influenced the development of medicine.

THE LEGEND OF CHINA'S FU XI AND NUWA

In *The Flood Myths of Early China,* Mark Edward Lewis relates the story of Fu Xi and NuWa (also NuGua), two semi-mythical spiritual progenitors representing yin and yang essence. The legend describes them as brother/sister and husband/wife, who repopulated the Earth after the primordial deluge, fashioning humans out of clay (wet earth), and teaching them hunting, fishing, cooking, and writing. NuWa, in particular, was said to have been the creator of humans an important distinction as we compare this account with Sumerian texts.[5] Cosmologist Laird Scranton supports Lewis's account, adding that the prevailing view of Chinese scholars is that Fu Xi was the first of eight ancestors, traditionally paired with NuWa, *nu* meaning "wife," and *fu* meaning "husband."[6]

Fu Xi's reign is generally accepted to have transpired in the third millennium BCE, and credited retrospectively for initiating Taoism, although Taoism was formulated much later. The origins of myths are difficult to pinpoint exactly since oral tradition extends much further back in history than do written texts. Varying accounts are inevitable, as are ambiguous timelines. What is consistent is the description of Fu Xi and NuWa as male and female deities that repopulated the Earth after a flood. Chinese history includes many floods throughout the ages (as in fact did occur), not just what can be associated with the Biblical flood, and the legends of Fu Xi and NuWa are associated with each one as a primal couple who protected their progeny—the human race.[7]

Several semi-mythical, semi-divine leaders and historic Chinese emperors are credited with eventually bringing the waters and floods under control, by constructing massive irrigation and flood control projects and creating canals for inland transportation. These historic developments are seen as central to the development of Chinese civilization and economy, and the organization and direction of labor in Chinese society.[8]

According to Lewis, the ancient art that depicts Fu Xi and NuWa is suggestive of an earlier version of the deities and their story, portraying them as having a male and female head with a serpent's body intertwining, as can be seen in figure 3.1. Recall that serpents and dragons were symbolically associated with deities across global cultures, perhaps going back hundreds of thousands of years, and that they balanced reproductive/kundalini energy and masculine/feminine energies for healing. The following quotation describes how this balancing led to cultural advancement.

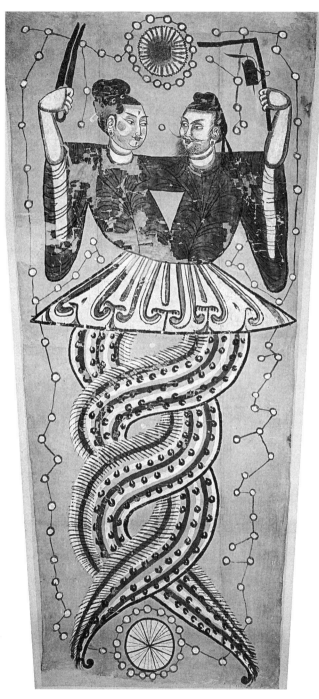

Fig. 3.1. Ancient painting of NuWa and Fu Xi
(also spelled "Fu Hsi") unearthed in Xinjiang.

In the beginning there was as yet no moral nor social order. Men knew their mothers only, not their fathers. When hungry, they searched for food; when satisfied, they threw away the remnants. They devoured their food, hide and hair, drank the blood, and clad themselves in skins and rushes. Then came Fu Hsi and looked upward and contemplated the images in the heavens, and looked downward and contemplated the occurrences on earth. He united man and wife, regulated the five stages of change, and laid down the laws of humanity. He devised the eight trigrams in order to gain mastery over the world.[9]

Author Eva Wong grew up in Hong Kong in the middle years of the twentieth century listening to the traditional tales of local storytellers, which were uncensored (by the Communists) chronicles called the *yeshi*. Her tale of Fu Xi begins:

After heaven and earth separated, yin and yang copulated. From this copulation countless myriad things emerged . . . Those that contained more of the essence of stillness became trees, grasses, and roots; those that contained more of the essence of movement became birds, mammals, fishes . . . those that contained more of the essence of spirit became humans . . . Thousands of years passed. The Early Ancient Era passed into the Middle Ancient Era, which in turn passed into the Later Ancient Era. In the Later Ancient Era there lived a sage named Fu Xi. Legends say that Fu Xi had a man's head and a snake's body. He taught the people hunting, fishing, animal husbandry and writing . . . he studied the paths of the sun, moon, and stars . . . examined the patterns of the mountains, lakes, and rivers. Finally he pondered the nature of the wind, rain, and thunder. . . . Fu Xi concluded that there are eight fundamental building blocks of the natural world . . . He named them the bagua, or the eight trigrams . . . "[10]

Laird Scranton corroborates the previous descriptions of Fu Xi as the one credited with "discovering" the eight trigrams of I Ching and, as mentioned above, for being one of the first of eight ancestors.[11] However, in terms of cosmology, accounts that allude to eight ancestors are not restricted to China. Egyptian texts also include Eight Primordials called the Ogdoad (or Ennead).

EGYPTIAN COSMOLOGICAL MYTHS

Two different myths in Egypt relate to Creation, perhaps because there are two primordial couples: Ptah and Sekhmet, god/goddess of Upper Egypt, and Khnumn and Neith, god/goddess of Lower Egypt.[12] Scranton relates the Egyptian Neith to the Chinese NuWa, as both are associated with biological reproduction and the primordial womb from which all life sprang.[13]

Egyptian oracle authors Athon Veggi and Alison Davidson describe Neith as "one of the ancient deities that predated the rise of the great Egyptian dynasties."[14] Her name comes from *Netet,* which means "weaver." Egyptian texts refer to her magical powers in mating energies that create new life, and describe her as one who possessed both male and female energies. She is credited for giving birth to the Sun god Ra (Marduk) and subsequently all other life.[15] Her Lower Egyptian counterpart Khnumn was known as the "Builder of Men, Maker of the Gods, the Father from the Beginning . . . " and described as one who molded the first human out of the mud of the Nile, "like a potter working with his wheel."[16] This description is congruent with Fu Xi as the male counterpart who "fashioned man out of clay."

According to ethno-psychologist Chris Hardy, Ph.D., author of *The DNA of the Gods,* the term meaning "clay" in Sumerian, and the term meaning "mud" in Akkadian refer to a woman's egg, another important distinction to remember as we continue.

ANCIENT SUMER'S ENKI AND NINMAH

In ancient Sumerian texts, another god/goddess couple is credited for populating (and re-populating) the Earth, with characteristics similar to Chinese Fu Xi and NuWa. Chris Hardy explains that while we use the term *Creator*, which connotes that humans were "made from scratch," Sumerian tablets use a verb meaning "to fashion" or "to perfect."[17] The Sumerian Creation story, as described on clay tablets discovered in Mesopotamia that date back to 3500 BCE, can be considered to describe interactions between humans and ancient groups referred to as the Anunnaki.

According to this story, the Annunaki needed gold to repair the atmosphere of their home planet, Nibiru, and set about mining it on Earth. Nibiru is a planetary body whose immense elliptical orbit cycles near Earth every thirty-six hundred years and would have theoretically crossed the terrestrial solar system during the time the Sumerian civilization existed. However, there now exists evidence of civilizations in South Africa hundreds of thousands of years before Sumer, which have also been linked with Nibiru.

The legend states that there came a time when the Annunaki miners rebelled and decided to fashion humans for the task instead. Ninmah was the head scientist, and was in charge of health matters for the Anunnaki. She was also put in charge of cultivating Earth's plant life with seeds she had brought with her for the purpose of producing medicinal plants. Through her work, agriculture, farming, and animal domestication advanced exponentially, as did an "Earth version of the Elixir of Immortality."[18] More important to the Creation story of man, Ninmah was commissioned to create a hybrid human: "Thus, Ninmah, daughter of Anu, through the vote in the Assembly, was assigned the 'perfecting' of a 'mixed creature'—a lulu—as a formal mission."[19]

Meanwhile, Enki had prepared a laboratory for Ninmah in Africa (Abzu), in Zimbabwe, near the mining center in South Africa. After much trial and error over a period believed to be about three hundred thousand years, "Adamu" was created, representing the first successful evolutionary attempt. The second leap in evolution was Tiamat, the first Earth-woman.[20] Hardy continues to explain that the ancient name for the region of Sumer was E.DIN, or Edin; it was located between the Tigris and Euphrates Rivers in Mesopotamia (Greek for "the land between rivers").

Ningishzidda, who according to Hardy was none other than

Hermes, son of Enki, performed the third evolutionary leap of human beings. Ningishzidda had been trained in Africa by Ninmah and in order to upgrade the DNA, he used both Ninmah's and Enki's DNA, which he extracted from their rib marrow.[21] It was this stage of evolution that elevated the self-consciousness of humans, their ability to think independently, and their ability to procreate—a goal that Enki and Ninmah had in mind for a long time.

Enki's brother Enlil, however, wanted to continue making clones to perform the mining operations, and took no interest in developing the human race as an intelligent, independent species.[22] According to the Sumerian tablets, this is what constituted the expulsion from E.DIN: 1) The first man and woman became aware of their sexuality, and 2) they were endowed with intelligence.[23]

How this relates to China's Creation myth and the importance of yin and yang in its medicinal tradition will be seen soon enough. For now, it is important to continue with the story of Enki and Ninmah as it leads to the origins of the Biblical Creation story as well as those of Egypt, Sumer, and South Africa.

Enki and Ninmah are described as advanced scientists who understood that Nibiru's demise was inevitable. They also knew that one of Nibiru's moons had originally seeded life on Earth, thereby having created DNA similar to theirs: "There had been an original collision of a moon of Nibiru (at that time a nomad planet) with the ancient huge planet called Tiamat that partly exploded, thus creating the asteroid belt . . . and the larger part being thrust into a new orbit nearer the sun, thus becoming our Earth. As for Nibiru, the planet was then captured by the gravitational field of our sun and started to orbit it. Enki realized why Earth life-forms and their DNA resembled that of Nibiru: life on Earth had been seeded by the original collision with Nibiru's moon."[24]

As the story continues, there developed an intensifying rivalry between Enki and his brother Enlil. Whereas Enki was responsible, along with Ninmah, for fashioning humans, Enlil saw them only as a means to an end—that of mining and obtaining precious metals for the reparation of Nibiru. It was he, upon discovering Adamu and Tiamat's "new consciousness" (that of being self-aware), who became enraged and cast them out of Edin. As the familiar text from Genesis states, "Behold the man is become as one of us . . . and now lest he put forth his hand and partake also of the Tree of Life, and eat, and live forever" (Genesis 3:22, King James Version). Using the term *one of us* implies that Enlil referred to the group of Anunnaki "royalty," from which the term *Elohim* stems, but contradicts the story of a singular God who rebukes Adam and Eve for becoming like Him. (The phrase "knowing good and evil" was excluded here on purpose since the ancient Sumerian texts contradict this phrase included in most modern translations of the Bible.) It also contradicts the previous warning to Adam and Eve (whether from a singular God, or Enlil for that matter) that they would die upon eating the fruit of the Tree of Knowledge.

In *DNA of the Gods,* Hardy states that on several Mesopotamian and Assyrian depictions there are two "astronauts" guarding the Tree of Life. She continues to explain that in the Epic of Gilgamesh, there is a description of Anu's Garden-Temple on Nibiru that had "two very special trees: The Tree of Knowing and the Tree of Life.[25] "The Tree of Life . . . was the tree bearing the fruit and from which (on Earth) both the Water of Life and the Bread of Life were made . . . these were the drink and food able to sustain longevity and to bestow a quasi-immortality to the Nibirians and the Anunnaki . . . The Tree of Knowing is represented . . . as referring to the genome bearing the DNA (the Essence of Life), with its pairs of bases (the symmetrical branches)."[26]

In Edin, Enlil asks Adamu, "Who told thee though that thou art naked?" His asking the question implies that he knows of another who is capable of imparting the (scientific) practices of the Anunnaki to Adamu and Tiamat. Just as Enlil became enraged by the deception of his "serpent" brother, which, by the way, was against Enlil, not Adamu and Tiamat, and which had enlightened the primitive workers (lulus) to their new "self-aware" status, Enlil also became incensed by their continued propagation.

While the Chinese Fu Xi and NuWa are not described as "extra-terrestrial," they are described as semi-divine celestial deities, and sometimes depicted as half-human, half-serpent. Sumerian texts show Enki as a deity with the lower body of a serpent and the upper body of a man

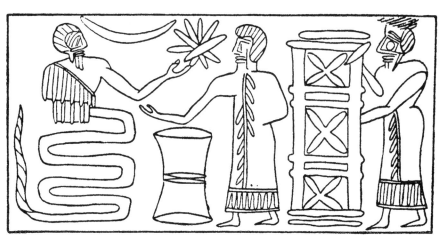

Fig. 3.2. Enki represented as a serpent-god imparting wisdom
to Ziasudra, warning of the coming flood.

who warns Ziusudra (Noah) of Enlil's intent to wipe out the human
race with the flood.[27]

These similarities have been analyzed by experts in comparative religion and archaeology, one of whom was Zecharia Sitchin (1920–2010),
who wrote: "As both Orientalists and Bible scholars now know, what
went on was the editing and summarizing by the compilers of the Book
of Genesis of much earlier and considerably more detailed texts written
down in Sumer."[28]

Sitchin endured much ridicule from the scientific/scholarly community during his lifetime, criticized for misinterpreting texts, astronomical information, and literalizing myth. Given that the church had
altered the word *mythos,* and other considerations, his interpretations
deserve a second look. Ongoing archaeological evidence is making
it more difficult to dismiss his work as "pseudo" history and science.
Perhaps some of the discrepancies that earned him criticism stem from
the fact that his conclusions may have been only partially true, but that
does not necessarily make them entirely false either.

Regarding the Biblical "Fall of Man," referring to the disobedience
of Adam and Eve, and the "Fall of the Angels," referring to the gods
who had relations with the "Daughters of Man," both served to ignite

Enlil's rage, who vowed to put an end to the whole species. Hardy quotes the text "'And the Lord said: I will destroy the earthling whom I have created off the face of the earth.'"[29] The text describes two attempts by Enlil to snuff out humanity, both of which failed due to Enki's interventions. The third attempt, by way of flood, succeeded, but Enki was able to save his son Ziasudra (Noah) and his family by instructing him to build a submersible vessel.[30]

Author, researcher, and scientist Michael Tellinger corroborates Sitchin's conclusions about the Anunnaki, making a distinction that Africa was the place of mankind's origin, and that Sumer came thousands of years later. His discoveries regarding the Dogon civilization of Africa suggest that the birth of terrestrial civilization originated two hundred thousand years prior to the tablets and hieroglyphs recorded in Sumer and Egypt.[31] These dates support Hardy's account that Abzu was the site of the first laboratory Enki set up for Ninmah and where she was able to teach Ningishzidda (Hermes/Thoth).

There is increasing evidence that supports the notion that many of Christianity's rituals, symbols, architecture, and doctrine were syncretically borrowed from, and based upon, original Sumerian and Egyptian texts. In *Return of the Serpents of Wisdom*, Pinkham writes about the Mesopotamian Anunnaki and the priest kings of Sumeria, Akkadia, and Babylonia, who were recognized as the messengers of Anu, "the great Spirit, and the vehicle of his serpent power on Earth . . . the rites and mantras practiced by these priests were believed to have been passed down from King Enmenduranki, the 'serpent king' of antediluvian Mesopotamia . . . part of the same lineage which produced the Egyptian Thoth-Hermes and the Hebrew Enoch."[32]

According to Richard Wilhelm and Cary Baynes, translators of the Chinese classic I Ching, Fu Xi was also thought to be the same as Enoch in the Bible.[33] All of these figures are described as those who became priests, ambassadors, scribes, teachers, and prophets. When we recall that Enoch was also a name ascribed to a "seer," prophet, priest, and scribe, the assignment to Fu Xi becomes plausible. Other parallels between this Chinese myth and ancient Sumerian texts as well as Egyptian accounts of Earth's post-flood repopulation can be found in the works of mythologist Joseph Campbell (1904–1987).

In *Oriental Mythology* Campbell lists the ten monarchs of early China, together with the ten Sumerian kings and the ten antediluvian patriarchs in the Bible, whose time periods all culminate with a great flood (see table 3.1). When we look at Dogon history, we discover a Creation myth even more ancient than these civilizations that shares similarities to China's cosmology.

TABLE 3.1. SUMERIAN, CHINESE, AND BIBLICAL CORRESPONDENCES

Sumerian Kings	Chinese Monarchs	Biblical Patriarchs
Alulim	Fu Xi and NuWa (NuGua)	Adam
Alagar	Shen Nung	Seth
Kidunnushakinkin	Yen Ti	Enosh
Eumengalanna	Huang Ti	Cainan
Divine Dumuzi	Shao Hao	Mahalel
Enmenluanna	Chuan Hsu	Jared
Eumenduranna	K'u	Enoch
Enzibzianna	Yao (Ti Yao)	Methuselah
Arad-gin	Shun	Lamech
Ziusudra	Yu (Yu the Great)	Noah

Source: Campbell, *Oriental Mythology*, page 119.

Please note that the figures in Campbell's list are not intended to describe actual history, as the chronology cannot be authenticated, but they do illustrate a pattern of correspondences among Sumer, China, and the Bible.

THE DOGON-CHINA LINK IN COSMOLOGY

In *The Cosmological Origins of Myth and Symbol,* Laird Scranton determines that we find the world's sole surviving hieroglyphic (or pictographic) language in China. Described as a priestly language, the

Na-khi-Dongba is named for the Dongba people. *Donga* is a word that means "sage," "shaman," "wise person," "sorcerer," and "teacher." Those who are familiar with the texts say that it "focuses on cosmological and religious subjects, including the formation of the universe and the world, and the processes of creation for all things, including humanity."[34]

Although Scranton admits finding no evidence that suggests direct contact between the Dogon and the Dongba, he believes that the Dongba are the Asian counterparts to the African Dogon. He references explorer, geographer, and linguist Joseph Rock (1894–1962) and Rock's book *The Ancient Na-khi Kingdom of Southwest China* in which Rock claims there were African influences on the Na-khi of China.[35]

One of the Dongba symbols for *na* takes the form of a loop and can be taken to indicate a manner in which primordial threads are woven into matter, referring back to the cosmological mother-goddess Neith who, as the Egyptian counterpart to the Dogon Nana (also Dada), weaves matter as well.[36] In China the Na-khi people are believed to be descendants of the nomadic tribe Qiang, who migrated through the valleys of northwest China, finally settling along the Jinsha River.[37] About three hundred thousand of them still exist in this region. They credit a group of revered ancestors for transforming them from nomads into a society by instructing them in the ways of metallurgy and farming, as is generally consistent with the classic Chinese accounts.[38]

Accepted as a sect of the Tibetan Bon religion, Scranton explains that Dongba cosmology conceives of the universe as being formed from a primordial egg. "Creation was associated with a great mother goddess whose symbol was a left-turning spiral."[39] One of the Na-khi Creation myths describes a magical incantation by which the power of the word replays and recreates the world. When we recall the Naacal tablets Joseph Churchward (1851–1936) helped translate, which refer to the mythical Mu, his findings are echoed by Scranton: " . . . the genealogy of the Dongba Mu ancestors (a term applied to the mythical founders of Dongba culture), like those of the Dogon is said to be linked to the creation of a cosmic order."[40] This correspondence could well be coincidence. Churchward's research took place in India, and with the relative proximity of India to China and Tibet, it's possible that the same Mu ancestors his research uncovered could also apply to the Dongba.

THE COSMIC EGG

Both Dogon and Dongba also describe the universe as being born by way of a cosmic egg with dual natures or paired opposites. Scranton says that the Dongba perceive their world as structured according to the east-west and north-south axes that are associated with the four cardinal points. They attribute the separation of earth and sky to an "incestuous marriage." While Scranton doesn't name the pair, the description is reminiscent of the brother/sister duo Fu Xi and NuWa. However, as per the Sumerian Creation story, it could also refer to the two original humans, Adamu and Tiamat, who were also brother and sister, and who also mated, inciting Enlil to eventually send a flood that would annihilate them. While purely speculative, this is consistent with the stories we've encountered to this point, given that Fu Xi and NuWa and Enki and Ninmah were described in the texts as protectors and teachers of the human race.

With regard to the four points, we find accounts associating NuWa with repairing the "four limits" responsible for holding up heaven, after damage by flood and fire. In one such account from the Huainanzi, China historian Mark Edward Lewis writes about in *The Flood Myths of Early China*.[41]

> In ancient times the four limits . . . collapsed and the Nine Provinces split apart. Heaven did not completely cover the world, nor did the earth support all things. Fires raged without going out, and water surged on without ceasing. Fierce beasts devoured the simple people, and birds of prey carried off old and young alike. Thereupon Nu Gua smelted the five-colored stones to patch the azure sky, cut off the turtle's legs to re-establish the four limits, and killed the black dragon to rescue Ji Province [the central of the Nine Provinces, which in this passage stands metonymically for the entirety of China]. She piled up ashes from reeds to halt the rampant waters.

Thus the azure sky was patched, the four limits corrected, the rampant waters dried up, Ji Province restored to order, and the treacherous creatures died. The simple people lived, walking on the back of the square provinces [fang zhou . . . the earth] and embracing the round Heaven.

CHAOS BEFORE THE CREATION

Just as NuWa is credited with restoring the four cardinal points that hold up heaven, so too did the sky goddess Nut in Egyptian lore. Nut bore the responsibility of protecting mankind from the forces of chaos (created by Set in Egyptian myth and Gong in Chinese myth). As shown in figure 3.3, Nut was portrayed as a naked woman covered with stars, whose hands/fingers and feet/toes touched the four cardinal points, thus forming the firmament above her husband, Geb (Earth).

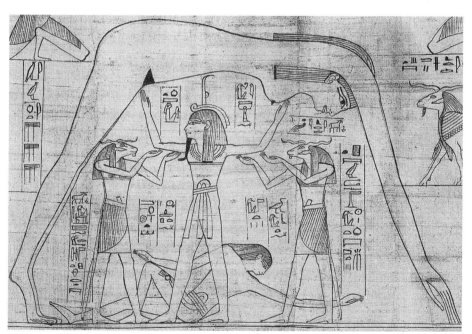

Fig. 3.3. A detail from the Greenfield Papyrus (*The Book of the Dead of Nesitanebtashru*). It depicts the air god Shu assisted by the ram-headed Heh deities, supporting the sky goddess Nut as the Earth god Geb reclines beneath. Photographed by the British Museum; original artist unknown.

In this scenario, separation of heaven and earth became necessary to restore and maintain order. Geb is also symbolized as an egg in Egyptian art.[42] In his book *The Cosmological Origins of Myth and Symbol,* Scranton explains that in the Dogon language *ogo* means "egg." We also recall that *mud* and *clay* in Chinese and Egyptian cultures translate to mean "egg" (also "womb"), and can see a common symbol underlying these ancient Creation myths.

THE EIGHT PRIMORDIALS

Veggi and Davidson describe the Egyptian Eight Primordials (also sacred Ogdoad), as a group of cosmic principles (or seed elements) from which the secret formation of matter is derived.[43] This conceptualization is similar to Eva Wong's description of Fu Xi's discovery of the Ba Gua, the eight trigrams of the I Ching: "eight fundamental building blocks of the natural world—sky, earth, water, fire, thunder, wind, mountain, and lake. Furthermore, these eight can be characterized by the way they embody and manifest the principles of yin and yang. He named them the bagua, or the eight trigrams . . . "[44]

The concept of the Chinese Eight Immortals can be understood if one accepts that the roots of later Taoism stretch far back into China's history, to the origins of shamanism. Shamanism includes the belief in a powerful spirit world that is inextricably connected to this world while also transcending it.[45] The word *Tao* means "way," as in "a way to know the truth." "Taoism offered the way of surrender to the ebb and flow of nature as the way to fulfillment."[46] The attitude of living apart from the material world and in harmony with nature can easily be seen in the stories of the Eight Immortals, who often resided in the mountains to practice meditation. Taoism, in its original expression, taught individuals how to achieve physical and spiritual immortality.[47] A quote from *The Yellow Emperor's Inner Canon* explains how living in harmony with the Tao delivers longevity: "I have heard that in ancient times there were the so-called Spiritual Men; they mastered the Universe and controlled Yin and Yang . . . They breathed the essence of life, they were independent in preserving their spirit, and the muscles and flesh remained unchanged. Therefore they could enjoy a long life, just as there is no end for Heaven and Earth. All this was the result of their life in accordance with Tao, the Right Way."[48]

In *Oriental Mythology,* Joseph Campbell quoted a professor of Taoism, Wing-tsit Chan (1901–1994), on Taoism's connection to alchemy, immortality, and astrology. (Recall that Fu Xi is credited for being the progenitor of Taoism.)

> Taoism . . . has a host of immortals and spirits, and a rich reservoir of . . . divination, fortune-telling, astrology, etc. It developed an elaborate system of alchemy in its search for longevity, which contributed much to material culture and scientific development in medieval China . . . It has often been associated with eclectic sects and secret societies and so has been an important element in a number of popular uprisings . . . However, its concentration on a good life on earth, its respect for both bodily and spiritual health, its doctrine of harmony with nature, its emphasis on simplicity, naturalness, peace of mind, and freedom of the spirit have continued to inspire Chinese art and enlighten Chinese thought and conduct.[49]

This description of Taoism is reminiscent of the Hermetic tradition outlined in the preceding chapter, its connection to alchemy, and the secret missions carried out by the Templars.

SHAMANIC ROOTS OF ALCHEMY

Mark Pinkham describes the Lung Dragons of China as a group of immortals. They were the Chinese Serpents of Wisdom associated with the heaven-dwelling winged dragon known as the Lung Dragon.[50] According to Pinkham, the earliest record of the Chinese Dragon Culture dates back to 4500 BCE, which is also around the time the ouroboros (later recognized as the benzene ring chemical structure) became known. A Neolithic (8000–6000 BCE) earthenware bust of a human with a snake moving up the spine to the top of the head suggests knowledge of kundalini energy. The first known members of this culture are believed to have lived in regions adjacent to the Kun Lun mountain range, in provinces now known as Hunan, Anhwei, and Szechuwan, and in a neighboring province now known as Shentung.[51]

Another name by which this group was called is Wu, whom Pinkham describes as "immortal magician priests . . . sorcerers, mediums, exorcists, rain makers, healers, alchemists and soul travelers with the power of disengaging their Dragon Bodies from their material sheaths and traveling inter-dimensionally at will. They were worshippers of Tai I, the supreme god which was the union of the polarity, yin and yang."[52] Pinkham adds that many Wu shamans were women, revered for their ability to channel heavenly wisdom and power while on Earth. Eventually the Wu multiplied into many different sects, with the medical wisdom being transferred to a group of Taoist doctors known as Sai Kung.[53]

According to Pinkham, Taoism was already a well-established religion prior to the widely accepted "modern Taoism" of Lao Tzu in 500 BCE, actually starting around 3000 BCE. His accounts suggest that, at the beginning of the golden age, lasting for approximately five hundred years, the various Dragon kingdoms became one cohesive empire, providing the impetus for an era of peace, wisdom, and a spirit of national unity.[54] He describes five mythical Dragon kings, descendants of the Lung Dragons, who became prominent: Fu Shi (Fu Xi) (circa 3000 BCE), Shen Nong (circa 2750 BCE), Huang Ti (circa 2650 BCE), Yao (circa 2350 BCE), and Shun (circa 2294 BCE), collectively representing the five elements (metal, wood, fire, water, and earth) in Chinese medicine.

Of the five Dragon kings, Huang Ti, also known as the Yellow Emperor, is perhaps the most famous to Westerners, and responsible for *The Yellow Emperor's Inner Canon,* a seminal medical text still prevalent in Chinese medical practice today. Representing the final and uniting phase/element, earth, he has historically been associated with the birth of Taoism, while Lao Tzu, in approximately 500 BCE, carried forth the Taoist religion.[55] According to traditional legend, Huang Ti was conceived by a ray of golden light that emanated to Earth from the seat of the Cosmic Dragon (the Big Dipper), and entered his mother's womb. He is said to have exhibited serpentine wisdom well beyond his years, speaking at only two months old, and mastering all of the sciences by the age of fifteen.[56] Most scholars date *The Yellow Emperor's Inner Canon* around 475–221 BCE. However, the work was not compiled until long after his death, approximately 100 BCE, while the Emperor himself is assigned much greater antiquity.[57]

These accounts offer some congruency with an alternate story about Jesus's death and resurrection being an Egyptian rite of passage that qualified him as the supreme Master Serpent of Wisdom. Consider his quote to the apostles to be "wise as serpents, and innocent as doves." In light of this information, as well as the Sumerian account of Enki and Enlil, it seems that (rather than defining the serpent as either good or evil) the ancients viewed it as a symbol representing the right use of power. The serpent came to symbolize learning how to transform a lower and less healthy state of being into a higher, wiser one. As with the ouroboros (like a serpent swallowing its tail), it represents the unceasing cycle of transformation beginning with life, proceeding into growth, waning into death, and returning back to life. These are the cycles the ancient Chinese believed to inextricably link heaven, earth, and humanity, as represented by the four seasons and five phases that translate to the physical body. In the *Tao Te Ching* (#42), it is written:

> *The Tao gives birth to One.*
> *One gives birth to Two.*
> *Two gives birth to Three.*
> *Three gives birth to all things.*[58]

One refers to the primordial egg (womb) or undifferentiated wholeness, two refers to yin and yang, three refers to heaven, earth, humanity, which then gives birth to all forms: In the beginning . . . was the primordial womb. With the womb was the primal and undifferentiated energy tumbling and swirling in the great chaos . . . This state of timeless time and spaceless space is called Wuji, the Limitless . . . out of the Limitless emerged . . . Peng Gu . . . Then yin and yang separated . . . the clear and weightless vapor rose and became heaven and the muddy and heavy vapor sank and became earth . . . all things were still intertwined . . . This state of inter-connectedness is called Taiji, the Great Limit . . . Millions of years passed . . . One day in his travels Peng Gu caught a glimpse of the Jade Maiden . . . Out of their union emerged the Emperor of the East and the Empress of the West . . . They are also known . . . as Father Wood and Mother Metal . . . gave birth to the Celestial Lord . . . the Celestial Lord gave birth to the Terrestrial Lord, and the Terrestrial Lord in turn gave birth to the Lord of Humanity. From these lords were born the myriad deities, the immortals, and the teachers of humanity.[59]

ASTRONOMY'S LINK TO YIN AND YANG

Now with the celestial origins and cosmological views of Chinese medicine described, we may begin to see how astronomy "weighs in" on the origins of yin and yang. When researching the origin of the yin-yang symbol, one discovers that when ancient astronomers observed the heavens, they measuring light and shadow as the sun made its apparent path around the earth through the year. In "A Geomedical Approach to Chinese Medicine: The Origin of the Yin-Yang Symbol," Stephen Jaeger states: "Its origin dates back at least 2500 years, probably much earlier, playing a crucial role in the for-mation of the Chinese ancient civilization."[60] While no one can say for sure how old this symbol is, Thomas Dietrich writes that Chinese astronomy dates back to 15,000 BCE: "Schlegel (1875) surmised from internal structural elements and the equinoctial and solstical positions that the Chinese maps of the heavens dated back to 15,000 BCE. In 1984, Julius Staal supported Schlegel's ideas."[61]

Figure 3.4 depicts a Chinese measuring pole, about 8 feet high, from which the ancient Chinese astronomers viewed the sky, recorded positions of the Big Dipper, and measured the shadow created by the Sun's movement to determine the four directions.

Sunrise is in the east, sunset in the west. The greatest light is in the south, at the point of the summer solstice, and is giving birth to

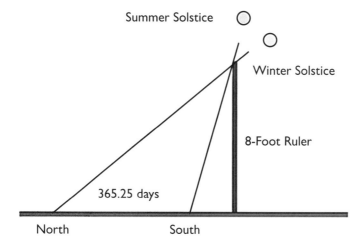

Fig. 3.4. Chinese measurement pole.
Source: http://chinesefortunecalendar.com/yinyang.htm.

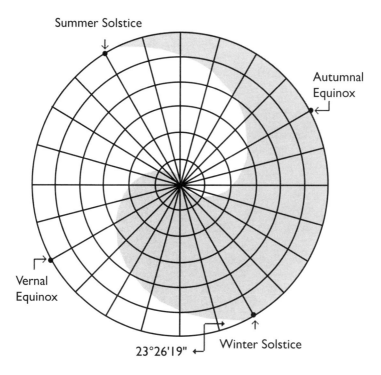

Fig. 3.5. Measurement of light and shadow reveal the yin-yang symbol.
Source: http://chinesefortunecalendar.com/yinyang.htm.

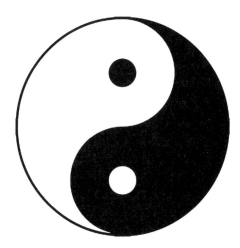

Fig. 3.6. Modern yin-yang (and I Ching) symbol.

shadow. In the north, at the point of the winter solstice, we have the longest shadow giving birth to light. The eight-foot-long pole, posted at a right angle to the ground, recorded the length of shadow and light, forming a circle with four seasons throughout the year.

Chinese astronomers then divided the circle of the year into segments, using six concentric circles around the pole, including the four cardinal points: vernal equinox, autumnal equinox, summer solstice and winter solstice, using the sunrise and Dipper positions (four angles × six circles = twenty-four segments). After connecting the points from summer solstice to winter solstice, a symbol such as the one in figure 3.6 was arrived at.[61]

AS ABOVE, SO BELOW

This information becomes more fascinating when one takes into account that there are, according to certain schools of thought, 365 acupuncture points on the body, coinciding with days of the year. There are twelve ordinary meridians, each assigned two hours in the twenty-four-hour period known as the circadian clock. There are also "pre-heaven" or extraordinary meridians (known as the eight extraordinary vessels) that correlate with the eight trigrams and the eight immortal beings.

Each acupuncture point is given a poetic name, signifying its spiritual purpose in addition to its physical one. For example, on the governing vessel (Du Mai), are points named Upper Star (GV-23) and Spirit Court (GV-24); on the kidney meridian, there is Spirit Seal (KI-23), Spirit Ruin (KI-24), and Spirit Storehouse (KI-25).[63] These are just a few examples that illustrate the inextricable link between healing of the physical body and the spiritual realm within the Chinese medical paradigm.

In the dated textbook, *Foundations of Chinese Medicine: A Comprehensive Text for Acupuncturists and Herbalists,* one finds a chart indicating the correspondences among the five element phases, organs of the body, and the planets.[64] This chart of correspondences is not taught in acupuncture schools today, but was part of the original system of Chinese medicine stemming from the Tao. Living in harmony with the Tao translated to living in a state of physical harmony within the body.

Huang Ti had his own semi-mythological doctor and medical minister (Qi Bo) with whom he conversed regularly. The structure of *The Yellow Emperor's Inner Canon* as a literary work is composed of a series of dialogues between the Yellow Emperor and his four ministers, of which one, Qi Bo, discusses medical issues. In the *Inner Canon* the Yellow Emperor is advised: "when the qi and shen are present and sound, no pathogen can invade a person, even when the cycles of nature are disruptive and plagues are near."[65]

The earlier semi-mythical Emperor Shen Nong (2750 BCE) was said to have been conceived when his mother "swallowed the vapor of a celestial dragon."[66] Shen Nong had a gift for understanding plants and herbs, and was always fascinated as a child by their healing properties. He is credited with compiling the original Chinese pharmacopeia estimated to have occurred in 1,000 BCE. It is said that one day he set out to learn from the herb master, but found a boy instead, who said the master had gone to the mountains to gather herbs, and could be gone anywhere from one week to one month. Determined to learn, Shen Nong set up his own hut. Seeing how determined he was, the boy entered into a kind of "Socratic" dialogue with him:

"Perhaps I can help you. What is it that you wish to learn?" Shen Nong said, "I'm puzzled by the fact that in ancient times people lived long and healthy lives but nowadays they get sick easily and often die before their time." The boy replied, "In ancient times people knew how to take care of themselves. They rose at sunrise and rested at sunset . . . they lived simply and had few desires. Knowing that it was better to prevent illnesses than to try to cure them, they ate healthy foods . . . And when they got sick, they knew how to apply the appropriate remedies. Today people hardly pay attention to their health: they don't eat properly, they don't rest sufficiently . . . they don't know the correct treatment . . . illnesses that can be cured easily often end up being serious or fatal."

Shen Nong then asked the boy how he could help people, and the boy gave him a book on the medicinal qualities of plants and told him to study, but said that if he really wanted to learn how to use them, he would have to experiment with them. When Shen Nong looked up the boy was gone. Shen Nong returned home and followed the advice of the boy by traveling, learning, identifying, and cataloging herbs, eventually creating a catalog of 365 medicinal plants. He taught the people how to farm properly, and how to protect plant habitats, "for if the places where the plants grow were destroyed, the science of herbal medicine would be lost to humanity forever."[67]

Whether myth, magic, or medicine is your preference, nature should be our priority and starting point. Only within nature will we find the answers we seek, whether spiritual or scientific. In the next chapter, we'll look at how the four elements comprise nature's building blocks, and provide the foundation for ancient cosmology and medicine.

4

THE FOUR BUILDING BLOCKS
OF THE COSMOS

Just as duality can be seen in every culture as a derivative of ancient astronomers' observations, so too do we find four elements that are fundamental to each. The twofold expression of yin and yang divides and becomes reflected in four expressions as moist-hot-dry-cold, spring-summer-autumn-winter, and birth-maturity-degeneration-death. In *The Culture of Astronomy*, Dietrich explains that these four elements pertain to cosmic law and are fundamental to the process of manifestation. The universe was formed in combinations of liquid, fire, gas, and solids—translating into the elements water, fire, air, and earth.[1]

The symbol or glyph used to depict the Earth is a circle with a cross in the center, as depicted in figure 4.1.

This symbol has also been used since antiquity to describe the

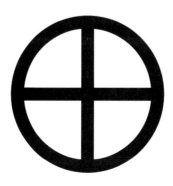

Fig. 4.1. Earth glyph symbol.

four directions, the four corners of the Earth, and the four angles in an astrology chart. In mathematics, geometry, and trigonometry it is known as the unit circle.

FOUR ELEMENTS IN
ANCIENT COSMOLOGY

In the previous chapter we presented the ancient Chinese legend that described Nu Gua as one who repaired the collapse of the four limits by patching them with her five-colored stones.[2] We also presented the Egyptian myth concerning Nut, which described her as one whose hands and feet touched the four corners of Earth, and whose star-covered body formed the heavenly firmament above Earth.[3]

NATIVE AMERICAN CULTURE

These four directions (and elements) are central to Native American myths as well. In *Star Ancestors,* Harriet Goodluck, a full-blooded Navajo elder, explains that her tradition divided the world into four: "We call these worlds Mother Earth (Nahas-tsan beh-assun), Father Sky (Yaah-diklith beh-hasteen), Holy Water (Toho), and Fire God (Hashjesh-jin) . . . When the world started it was the end of another world . . . Earth is still alive and Water is still making it live . . . All life goes back into a world far ahead of us. The balls of stars, the comets, are living messengers."[4]

Author Nancy Red Star quotes Chief Dan Katchonga from the Sun Clan of the Hopi Sovereign Nation whose tradition teaches about migration to the four regions of Earth: "The Hopi were survivors of another world that was destroyed. Therefore, Hopi were here first and made four migrations—North, South, East, and West—claiming all the land for the Great Spirit, as commanded by Massau, and for the True White Brother who will bring on Purification Day."[5]

Similar prophecies exist in the Cherokee tradition, which speak of ancient "scientists" (Star Ancestors) who came from heaven, rescued Indian people from the sinking Atlantis, and instructed them to migrate to America. These prophecies contradict historical versions that Indians came from Asia across the Bering Strait and into Alaska, instead saying that the migration took place via Mesoamerica after the sinking of Atlantis.

> We were rescued by the Star Nations, the Creator, the survivors landed in Mesoamerica, the birthplace of the last migration. That was the center, and from there we traveled the four directions—north, south, east, and west—building pyramidal monuments in each sector. In Tibet the great white pyramid was built in the Himalayan mountain range; in Cambodia, the pyramid of Angkor; in Egypt, the pyramid on the Giza plateau . . . Go to the Yucatan for the spring equinox. Stand at the Temple of Seven Powers and witness the dawn through the cosmic portal. You will see the full flourishing of our ancient culture there.[6]

The Cherokee believe that the Star Ancestors are here to help heal the four races, whom they identify with the four elements: " . . . The White race has forgotten . . . The responsibility of fire . . . The Black race has forgotten . . . The responsibility of water. . . . The Yellow race has forgotten . . .The responsibility of air . . . The Red race is losing . . . The responsibility for earth . . . the Earth is out of balance. . . ."[7]

FOUR ELEMENTS
IN ANCIENT RELIGION

In *The Secret Doctrine,* Madame Blavatsky wrote that in essence there is but one element at the root of which lies the Supreme Deity. "From this supreme element, expressions of the Deity form the other elements: Fire, Air, Water, Earth were but the visible garb, the symbols of the informing, invisible Souls or Spirits—the Cosmic gods to whom worship was offered by the ignorant . . . respectful recognition by the wiser."[8]

Blavatsky explained that the origin of the four elements is identical with representations in other nations, including Upper Egypt, Israel, and the Americas, stating that in each place all nature was embraced in unity. The four elements were no more or less important than their creations in the form of trees, rivers, mountains, and stars.[9]

Dietrich cites James Wasserman in *Art and Symbols of the Occult, Images of Power and Wisdom,* who says that religion defines the first principle of reality as contained, for example, in the Hebrew name IHVH (Jehovah), with each letter corresponding to one of the four elements.[10] In Hebrew, as in Arabic and Semitic languages, the consonants are written down without the vowels, thus, four letters as written becomes Jehovah when spoken—although care is taken with speaking the name.

In *Natural Magic* Cornelius Agrippa (1486–1535) wrote: "The only true name of God, according to the cabala, is the name of four letters—the Tetragrammaton—Yod-he-vau-he."[11]

According to Blavatsky, the name Jehovah combines masculine and feminine attributes: " . . . separating into man and woman, and becoming JAH-HEVA in one form . . . It is found in fable and allegory, in myth and revealed Scriptures, in legend and tradition. Because, of all the great Mysteries, inherited by Initiates from hoary antiquity, this is one of the greatest . . . The compound name of Jehovah, or Jah-Hovah, meaning male life and female life . . . for the Hebrew letter Jod was the membrum virile and Hovah was Eve, the mother of all living, or the procreatrix, Earth and Nature."[12]

As reflected in the four letters, another reference to the four elements and directions in the Bible can be found in Revelations 4:7 (King James Version), which speaks about the four living creatures who also correspond to the four astrological constellations of Leo, Taurus, Aquarius, and Scorpio: "The first creature was like a lion, and the second creature like a calf, and the third creature had a face like that of a man, and the fourth creature was like a flying eagle . . . "

Ancient art depicts how our ancestors divided the horizon into four quarters, assigning spiritual attributes to each and creating temples in similar fashion. The term *tetramorph* refers to such designs, stemming from the Greek words *tetra* ("four") and *morph* ("shape"). This practice is the likely reason why the mythical sphinx has these

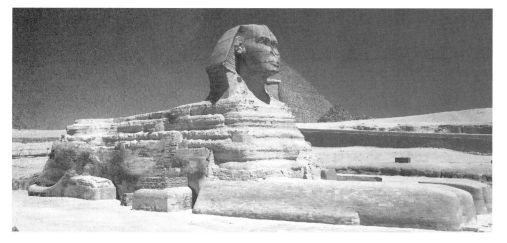

Fig. 4.2. Egyptian Sphinx. Photograph by Barcex (CC BY-SA 3.0).

four characteristics depicted in its visage: face of a human, feet of a lion, wings of the eagle, and body of the bull. In the Greek version all four elements were included, with the human face being that of a woman; the Egyptian Sphinx includes the face of a man believed to be that of Pharaoh Khafra (Fourth Dynasty, third millennium BCE), but excludes the eagle's wings.

Figure 4.3 shows the movement of the solstices and equinoxes throughout history. In *Sacred Number and the Origins of Civilization,* Richard Heath explains that over the twenty-six-thousand-year period known as the "Great Year," the equinoctial points shift: "The tilt of Earth's axis leads to the excursions of the Sun above and below the celestial equator . . . The precession of the pole over 26,000 years means that there is also a precession of these equinoctial points within the zodiac."[13]

There was a time approximately six thousand years ago, when the equinoctial points corresponded to the signs of Aquarius (man), Scorpio (eagle), Leo (lion), and Taurus (bull). Recall, as well, the verse from the Book of Revelations describing these beings as creatures that guard the gates of heaven. This tetramorph exists in Christian art, symbolizing the four Gospels of Christ as well as the four creatures and four elements.

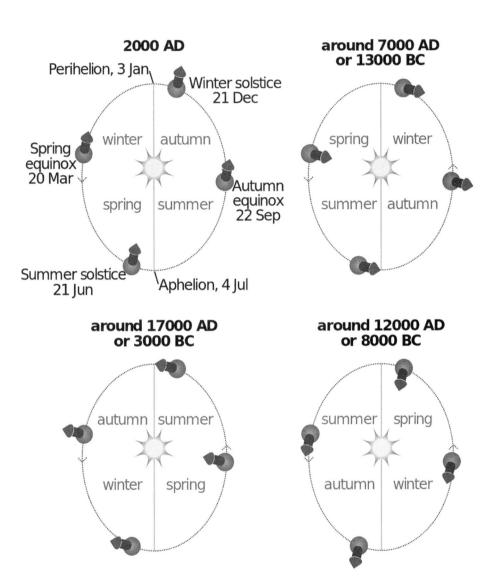

Fig. 4.3. The relationship between the apses, seasons, and precession of Earth's axis, viewed from north. The seasons pertain to the Northern Hemisphere and are reversed for the Southern Hemisphere. The tilt of Earth's axis and the eccentricity of its orbit are exaggerated. Illustration by Cmglee (CC BY-SA 3.0).

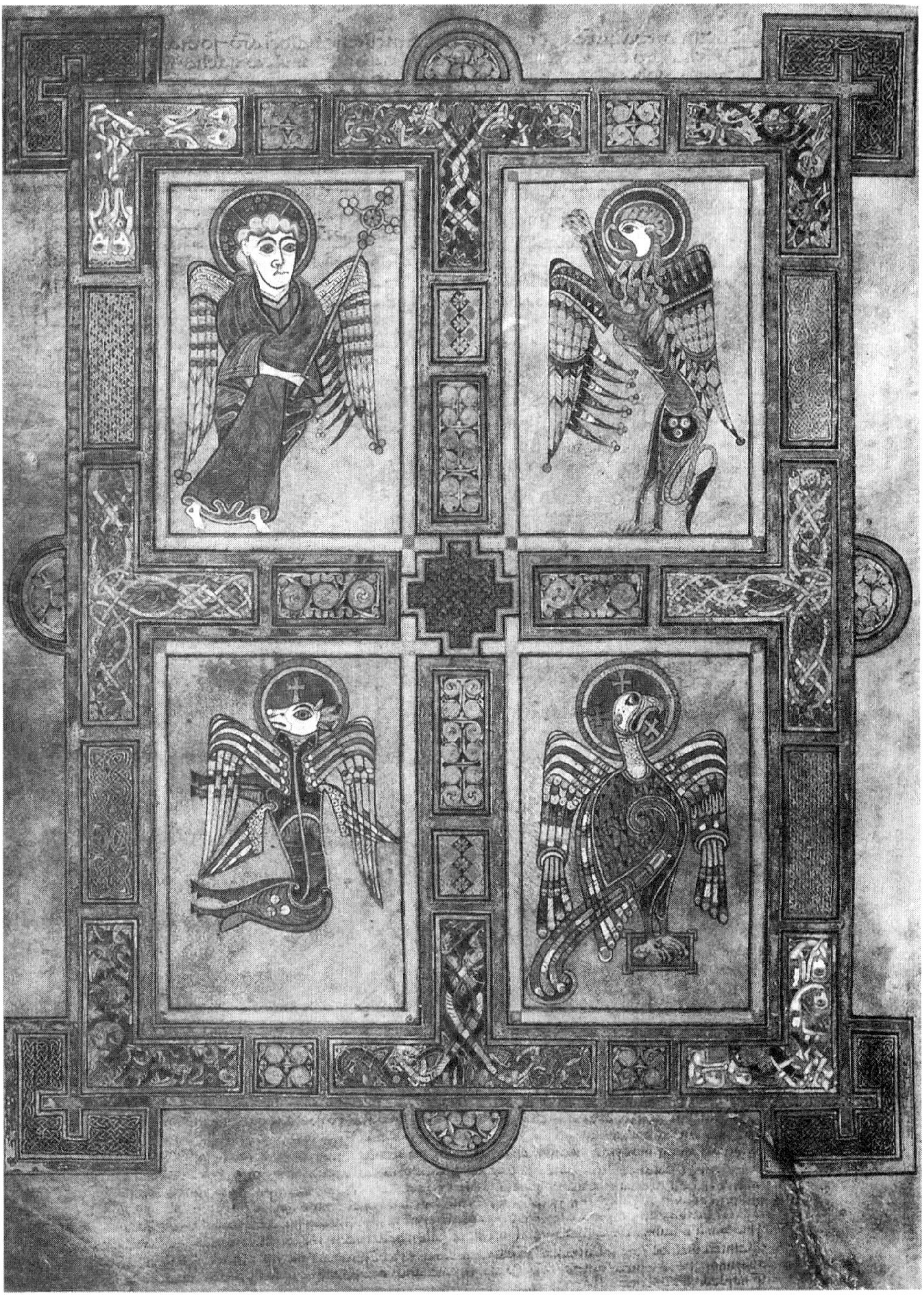

Fig. 4.4. The four evangelists, as illustrated in the Book of Kells
(an illuminated manuscript of Gospels in Latin), circa 800.

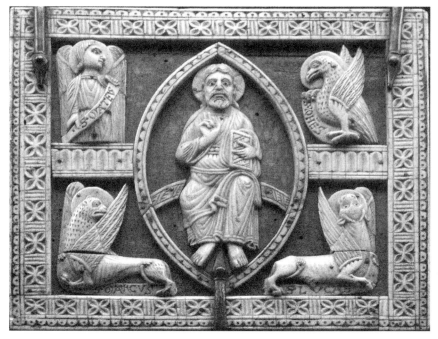

Fig. 4.5. A thirteenth-century Cluniac (French Benedictine monastic order) ivory carving of Christ surrounded by the creatures of the tetramorph. Photograph by Marsyas (CC BY-SA 3.0).

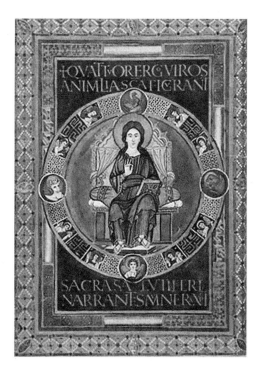

Fig. 4.6. Folio 72 verso from the Lorsch Gospels (circa 778–820) depicting Christ in majesty.

In correlating the four elements to alchemy, Eliphas Levi (1810–1875) explains that they are known as salt, sulphur, mercury, and azoth (first principle of all metals):

> Here let us add a few words on the four magical elements . . . in alchemy, Salt, Sulphur, Mercury and Azoth; in hieroglyphics, the Man, Eagle, Lion and Bull; in old physics . . . air, water, earth and fire. But in magical science we know that water is not ordinary water, fire is not simply fire, etc. . . . Modern science has decomposed the four elements of the ancients and reduced them to . . . simple bodies. That which is simple however, is the primitive substance . . . there is thus only one material element, which manifests always by the tetrad in its forms. We shall therefore preserve the wise distinction of elementary appearances by the ancients, and shall recognize air, fire, earth and water as the four . . . visible elements of Magic . . . To these four elementary forms correspond the four . . . philosophical ideas: Spirit, Matter, Motion, Rest . . . which alchemy has reduced to three—the Absolute, the Fixed and the Volatile—referred by the Kabala to the essential idea of God. . . .[14]

Levi is saying that the elements are symbolic, and are understood as visible evidence of what alchemists call magic and religious/spiritualists call God. And so even while at certain points in time the equinoctial points have fallen into different constellations, this positioning is less important than understanding them as ideas. It will also be important to remember the reduction of four elements into three principles— absolute, fixed, and volatile—when we discuss astrology a little later.

FOUR ELEMENTS IN TAROT

The same four elements can also be found in both playing cards and Tarot divination cards. Incidentally, Tarot (also Taro) itself comes from the Kabbalistic tetragram representing the four elements.[15] A regular deck of cards is comprised of the suits of hearts, spades, clubs, and diamonds (water, fire, air, and earth).

In Tarot decks, we have cups, wands, swords, and pentacles. Hearts and cups represent water/emotional experience, spades and wands represent fire (soul, spirit, spiritual growth/initiation) encompassing, infusing, and informing all aspects of life. Swords and clubs represent mental activity—words act like swords to cut through emotion and make a logical decision; clubs represent mental focus and concentration, often writing and communicating also. Finally, there is earth, representing material resources with diamonds (precious gems discovered deep in the earth), and pentacles (coins/material possessions). These elements are a part of our everyday life, yet we may not always realize this connection.

It's important to note as well that Tarot has no "birth" card, only a "death" card. This circumstance is not for the purpose of emphasizing morbidity; rather it is meant to emphasize the need for change and transformation that ultimately results in birth. If drawing of the death card is taken literally, it creates fear and panic in the individual. It could refer to an actual death, but more often than not, it merely refers to significant change, ultimately leading to something new (spring). Anytime we humans face change, whether the loss of a loved one, loss of a job, or an unwanted disease/diagnosis, we tend to feel that the effects are devastating and permanent, failing to remember the temporary nature of such experiences.

FOUR ELEMENTS IN THE CROSS

One of the oldest and best-known religious symbols is the cross. About the cross, Blavatsky states that its original meaning was one having to do with the mysteries of initiation, not crucifixion.

> The initiated adept, who had successfully passed through all the trials, was attached, not nailed, but simply tied on a couch in the form of a Tau of a Swastika without the four additional prolongations, plunged in a deep sleep (the "Sleep of Siloam" it is called to this day among the Initiates in Asia Minor, in Syria, and even higher Egypt). He was allowed to remain in this state for three days and three nights, during which time his Spiritual Ego was said to confabulate with

the "gods," descend into Hades, Amenti, or Patala (according to the country), and do works of charity to the invisible beings, whether souls of men or Elemental Spirits; his body remaining all the time in a temple crypt or subterranean cave. In Egypt it was placed in the Sarcophagus in the Kings Chamber of the Pyramid of Cheops, and carried during the night of the approaching third day to the entrance of a gallery, where as a certain house the beams of the rising Sun struck full on the face of the entranced candidate, who awoke to be initiated by Osiris, and Thoth, the God of Wisdom.[16]

This description is consistent with what was discussed in chapter 1 concerning Mark Amaru Pinkham's alternate theory about Christ's death and resurrection. Gerald Massey (1828–1907), Egyptologist, English poet, and controversial author, offered a theory that Jesus's life, as depicted in the Christian scriptures, reflects the four-phased birth-growth-degeneration-death cycle with his birth, betrayal, Crucifixion, and Resurrection. This cycle is also reflected in the four phases of the moon. At the new moon, when the moon conjuncts the sun, there is a new cycle (birth). When the moon waxes to the first quarter phase, there is growth. When the moon opposes the sun and reaches its fullness, there is crossing over immediately into darkness (crossification). It continues to wane and die, that is, it becomes completely dark at the time of the new moon when the cycle repeats (resurrects the light).

An objective of this book is to show astronomical correlation to all systems, including religion. In this spirit I share Massey's findings on the subject from his book *The Historical Jesus, and the Mythical Christ.*

According to the synoptics, Christ died on the 15th of the month of Nisan, but in John's narrative the crucifixion occurs on the 14th of Nissan. . . Thus a death of the Christ on Thursday and a resurrection on Saturday were continued alongside of a crucifixion on Friday and the rising again on Sunday. Now, the date assigned for the crucifixion is determined by the full moon of Easter . . .But there were two different dates for the full moon . . . Here then is a natural genesis for the two traditions of the crucifixion (passover or crossing) that was reputed to have occurred on the 14th and on the 15th of the month.[17]

In other words, Easter, the time of Christ's passion and resurrection is not observed on a set date, but always falls on the first full moon after the vernal equinox. Massey's point is that if there were an actual historical date for this event, the date would remain consistent each year; this circumstance is similar to Passover as well. (And, of course, all actual dates changed from the Augustinian to the Gregorian calendar back in history.)

With regard to the cross and the Kabbalistic Tetragram, Eliphas Levi explains

> The four astronomical cardinal points are . . . manifestations of the First Cause . . . revealed invariably by the Cross—that unity made up of two, divided one by the other in order to produce four; that key to the mysteries of India and Egypt. The Tau of the patriarchs, the divine sign of Osiris, the Stauros of the Gnostics, the keystone of the temple, the symbol of Occult Masonry, the Cross, central point of the junction of the right angles . . . seems to be the first root and fundamental substantive of the verb to believe and the verb to grow, thus combining the conceptions of science, religion and progress.[18]

The *Catholic Encyclopedia* also observes that the cross was a symbol used long before the time of Christ, and thus is not unique to it. "The sign of the cross, represented in its simplest form by a crossing of two lines at right angles, greatly antedates in both the East and West to the introduction of Christianity. It goes back to a very remote period of human civilization."[19]

With regard to making the sign of the cross, Levi explains that the "occult" version of the Paternoster (the Our Father) included two ways of making the sign of the cross, one for initiates and the other for non-initiates, with its original meaning representing "the oppositions and quarternary equilibrium of the elements." The initiates would say "To thee belong," while their hand was at their forehead, "the kingdom," while carrying the hand to the chest, "justice" while taking the hand to the left shoulder, "and mercy" as the hand was moved to the right shoulder.[20]

In the pre-Christian era even the swastika was a symbol depicting the four elements (and found in both Sanskrit/Indian and Native American/Indian depictions, for example). As such, it has nothing to do with its modern-day association with the twentieth-century German National Socialist regime. This unfortunate association provides a dramatic example that some ancient symbolic meanings can change according to cultural perceptions.

Not only does the cross reflect the four directions, so too do the number of Gospels in the Bible (according to Iraneus): "The Gospels could not be either more or less in number than they are, as there are the four zones of the world via which we all live."[21]

In the astrological system we know as "Western" or "tropical" astrology, it is again the four elements we find at the foundation of its interpretation. Before we delve into these characteristics, we will address the general contrast between Eastern and Western points of view.

THE SYMBOLIC SKY

In *Astrology Decoded* international lecturer and instructor at the London School of Astrology, Sue M. Farebrother, explains that the zodiac circle was identified by ancient astrologers and divided into twelve equal parts. Almost all systems of astrology use these twelve zodiac signs. However, determining what constellations are used for the planets is where East and West differ. In East Indian Vedic (or sidereal) astrology, charts are based upon the literal placement of the stars, which are much further away from Earth than are the planets, and have unequal divisions (anywhere from 9° to greater than 30°). It is also a system that arose from, and is based upon, the Hindu caste system, which tends to have a more fatalistic perspective of one's life.[22] In the tropical system, interpretation is based upon an equal division of the 360° circle, giving each sign 30° and lasting approximately a month. (Please note that this is different from the precessional cycle in which the Earth's pole moves backward through the zodiac circle at a rate of 2,160 years per constellation—known as an age. The sun, from our perspective, moves about 1° per day or 30° per month.)

Interpretations based on Western astrology lend more flexibility in terms of a person's free will in responding to planetary influences. They are also based upon the monotheistic worldview predominant in the West, which we have discussed in preceding chapters insofar as the sun (godhead) is at the center of the twelve expressions of our solar system traveling with it through space. (Fig. 4.7 provides a

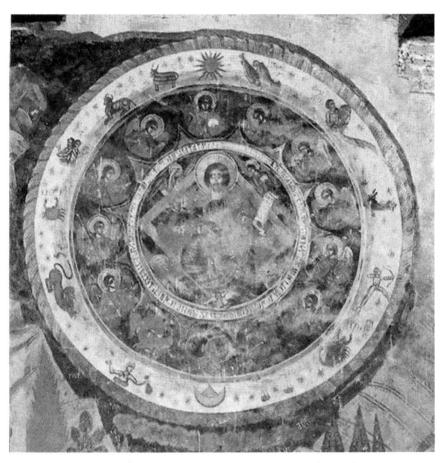

Fig. 4.7. A fragment of a seventeenth-century fresco from Svetitskhoveli Cathedral in Mtskheta, Georgia, depicting the zodiac with Christ at the center.

seventeenth-century depiction of the Christ-centered zodiac.) Since we live in a "solar system," the Western version of astrology bases its perspective on the sun—hence the measurement of light through the four seasons, elements, and expressions. The astrological chart, however, is drawn from the geocentric viewpoint, taking a snapshot of the heavens from the specific latitude/longitude of the place on Earth at the moment a person is born.

As one who encourages individual choice as well as a scientific attitude of exploration, I offer readers my contributions, which are based upon personal experience and combined with current knowledge and a curiosity guided by intuition. I have always found Western astrology to be profoundly accurate as well as a constant source of inspiration.

That is not to say that Vedic or other astrological systems such as Chinese or Native American would not be equally relevant and inspirational. When it comes to taking up the study of self, I am in favor of individuals coming to that decision on their own, seeking guidance from experts of their choosing as they feel the need. Because Western astrology is the more fluent language for me, that will be my focus for this discussion.

The circle divided by two polarities is expressed as masculine (yang) and feminine (yin). Yin and yang divide to become four elements, and also correspond to the four directions. Fire and air are placed along the east-west axis, representing yang energy. Earth and water are placed along the north-south axis, representing yin energy. In addition to this directional correspondence, the four elements also connect with our four seasons, as stated, regarding the equinoctial points: fire aligns with the vernal equinox (spring) in the sign of Aries, with the air element taking its opposite place at the autumnal equinox (fall) in the sign of Libra. Earth is associated with the winter solstice and the sign of Capricorn, with water in its opposite placement at the summer solstice in the sign of Cancer (depending on whether one lives in the northern or southern hemispheres, the solstices will be experienced opposite each other; winter in the north will be summer in the south).

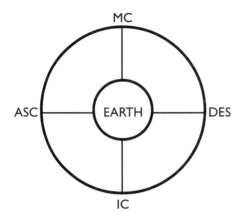

Fig. 4.8. Four angles in a horoscope chart. ASC (Ascendant) represents the sign rising in the east at the time a person is born. This is where Aries sits in the "natural zodiac" chart.

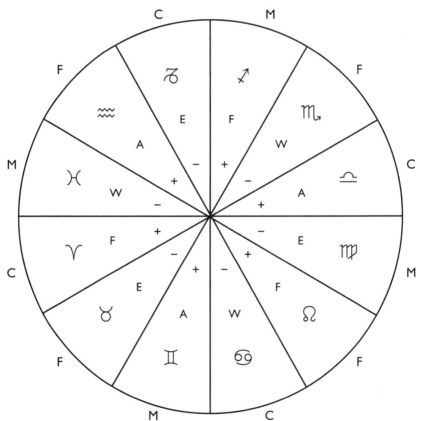

Fig. 4.9. Natural Zodiac Chart: beginning with Aries in the east, vernal equinox position. Shows the elements (FEAW: fire, earth, air, water); modes (CFM: cardinal, fixed, mutable), and yang (+ sign) or yin (– sign) indicators.

CHARACTERISTICS
OF THE FOUR ELEMENTS

When we consider how these elements operate in the physical realm, albeit in their extreme and primitive expressions, we can more easily understand how they behave psychologically in individuals. Fire and air are yang elements, and are characterized by upward active motion (smoke rises, air lifts). Earth and water are yin elements, and are characterized by downward, more receptive qualities (plants grow roots deep into the earth, and water soaks into the earth).

Yang elements like to move quickly. Fire in the extreme consumes anything in its path and transforms it. It can be noisy, roaring with a vengeance, and is difficult to control (highly impulsive and combustive). Air, in its extreme expression, can decimate an entire community, inflicting chaos in very short order, as with tornados and hurricanes. Air is impossible to pin down. It has no roots and prefers to keep circulating.

The challenge for yang elements is to slow down long enough to connect and process, which are yin qualities. For instance, when fire is able to slow down, it interacts rather than overpowers, which allows a more balanced transformation to take place. Physiologically, fire manifests as a fever, which purifies (burns off) pathogens and toxins that invade the body. The air temperament's challenge is to settle down—to practice grounding itself on the earth and being present in the body, rather than processing situations from a strictly intellectual point of view. Air's healing gift is its uplifting quality, which is needed when emotions become too heavy, or the body becomes too stagnant, lacking circulation and movement. Its objectivity and humor are refreshing in situations that feel too intense.

In contrast to the quick moving yang elements, earth and water involve a slower process. From our perspective, earth is unchanging and immoveable. It may be moving along in space with the entire solar system, but from where we stand—literally—it is stable. In its extreme, the earth temperament is adversarial to change, especially with regard to emotional and spiritual responses. Believing largely in the tactile world of the five senses, it has difficulty relating within emotional or spiritual connections because they are intangible. The key word for earth is *pragmatism;* however, *s*ome situations require intuition. Physiologically, the earth element sustains us through our food consumption and the metabolic processes. The earth temperament's gift is creating safety, stability, security, and dependability.

Water certainly moves, but unless exacerbated by extreme weather involving all of the elements, its process is also a slower one. It takes time for water to erode the environment. In water, we also witness the process of bonding, whereby it takes on the shape of its surroundings. It is impossible to distinguish one drop of water from the rest of the ocean, lake, or river, and that body of water takes on the shape of the surrounding earth basin. So for people with a water temperament, it is extremely difficult to separate from the environment in which they find themselves, especially regarding emotional responses. They automatically feel at one with those around them, evoking a very intangible but deeply felt connection, positive or negative. The extreme of the water temperament, then, finds it challenging to extricate itself from unwanted attachments, whether a person or situation. Physiologically, water nourishes us, supports metabolic and neurological processes, and connects and conducts energy. The healing characteristic of the water temperament is empathy, connection, and compassion.

None of these four expressions is superior to the other, as each one balances out its opposite and the other three expressions. Likewise, within the context of maintaining individual health, all four elements need to stay in equilibrium. The same holds true for planet Earth, whose extremes we experience as drought, flooding, freezing, or heat.

Now that we've looked at the zodiac circle divided by two polarities and four elements we will introduce another division based upon triplicity. Each of the four elements has within it three expressions called *modes,* which correlate to the three different signs belonging to each element. While I have not found information to support that these modes correspond to the absolute, fixed, and volatile principles mentioned above regarding alchemy, it is a curious coincidence nonetheless.

CARDINAL, FIXED, AND MUTABLE

Cardinal signs add a quality of initiating or catalyzing the element. Fixed signs tend to harness, to draw in the element. Mutable signs will want to change the element or make an adjustment in some way. To apply the idea, we will use Aries as an example. Aries is cardinal fire, so one could say that they are desirous of "starting a fire" (being argumentative), being impulsive, if their temperament is not self-contained or evolved. Aries rules the head, and so they are often seen as being headstrong.

TABLE 4.1. NATURAL ZODIAC CHART TABLE

Houses	Element	Mode	Zodiac Sign	Polarity
1st	Fire	Cardinal	Aries	Yang (+)
2nd	Earth	Fixed	Taurus	Yin (-)
3rd	Air	Mutable	Gemini	Yang (+)
4th	Water	Cardinal	Cancer	Yin (-)
5th	Fire	Fixed	Leo	Yang (+)
6th	Earth	Mutable	Virgo	Yin (-)
7th	Air	Cardinal	Libra	Yang (+)
8th	Water	Fixed	Scorpio	Yin (-)
9th	Fire	Mutable	Sagittarius	Yang (+)
10th	Earth	Cardinal	Capricorn	Yin (-)
11th	Air	Fixed	Aquarius	Yang (+)
12th	Water	Mutable	Pisces	Yin (-)

On the positive side, they are natural pioneers, great at getting projects started, and taking action to get it done. They are the quintessential "let's do it" people of the zodiac.

Taurus is fixed earth, so one could describe this combination as drawing in material resources, or harnessing Earth's energy in some way, perhaps through gardening or conservation. As an archetype ruled by Venus, Taurus individuals love the fine arts and/or the art of beautifying the environment or their home (a material possession). The modes go around the zodiac starting with Aries, in the order of cardinal, fixed, mutable, and repeat four times throughout the circle (three modes times four elements is equal to twelve signs of the zodiac). Elements go around the zodiac in the order of fire, earth, air, water, and repeat three times throughout the circle (four elements times three modes is equal to twelve signs of the zodiac).

NATURAL ZODIAC VERSUS NATAL CHART

The natural chart is different from the natal chart (birth chart of individuals). The natural chart is shown in figure 4.9 (page 86). It describes

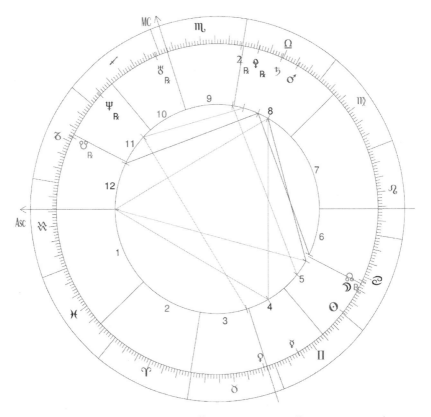

Fig. 4.10. Natal chart showing a different sign/constellation rising in the east so that the angles differ from the natural chart.
Source: "Natal Chart—Adam" by Morn (CC BY-SA 3.0).

the geocentric orientation to the four seasons, directions, and elements.

The natal chart represents a snapshot of the heavens at the moment an individual is born. Even if two people are born at the exact time and place, thereby sharing the same snapshot so to speak, their individual levels of consciousness influence how and to what extent they are able to work with and express the energies inherent in their chart.

The moment of birth is significant because it represents what might be referred to as the "celestial signature," or "cosmic imprint." In tropical astrology, it is the cardinal signs we find on the axes of the natural horoscope chart. Aries-Libra (east-west, ASC-DES), and Cancer-Capricorn (south-north, MC-IC). (Please refer to figs. 4.8 and 4.9 on page 86.) As already mentioned, this orientation is based upon the spring equinox (March 21), which is Earth's cycle. Obviously not everyone is born on March 21, and natal charts will all look different from the natural. However, the meanings of the angles, consistent with the elements, still hold true: east/asc/self, south/MC/outer world, west/desc/other, and north/IC/inner world.

There is much within a natal chart that can lead to better self-understanding and self-awareness. When you take into consideration that within the basic framework of the polarities, angles, elements, and modes, we also have the mathematical placement of the planets in their signs, expressing energy in an area of life (or house), there are multidimensional variables to consider. I encourage those who are interested to seek the help of a professional astrologer in deciphering one's chart. The objective here is to focus on the elements as we find them expressed in the physical realm and, specifically, to determine how they may be used as a tool for medicinal application.

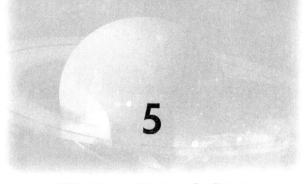

5

THE HEXAGON PHENOMENON

The real voyage of discovery consists not in seeking new lands but seeing with new eyes.

MARCEL PROUST

The Hermetic teaching "As above, so below," although an esoteric philosophy, is also a universal principle found in nature. When we explore the ancient arts and sciences we are witnessing a system designed to awaken our perception and trigger our memory. At the same time, repeating patterns found in nature gently coax us out of the illusion of separation and guide us back to connection. All aspects of nature, including the human anatomy, support reconciliation between the microcosm and macrocosm. From a distance our eyes take in the panoramic view, often missing the inner landscape. The quote "Can't see the forest for the trees" becomes "Can't see the trees for the forest." Neither view is better given that they each offer an important and unique perspective on the connectedness of life.

We explored the four elements in the last chapter. In this chapter, we will take a closer look at the significance geometry plays in micro and macro nature. Specifically, from the water element there are two very fascinating examples of microscopic patterns that are the work of Wilson A. Bentley (1865–1931) and Dr. Masaru Emoto (1943–2014).

THE SECRET LIFE
OF SNOWFLAKES

Wilson A. Bentley was born in Jericho, Vermont, on February 7, 1865. As a teenager growing up on a farm and exposed to long winters, he became interested in snow crystals. At first he tried to draw what he was seeing through the microscope his mother had given him, but the snow crystals were too complex to capture before they melted. Once able to purchase and attach a bellows camera to the microscope, he was able to photograph the crystals, but still endured many years of trial and error before finally succeeding in capturing his first snowflake image on January 15, 1885. "Under the microscope, I found that snowflakes were miracles of beauty; and it seemed a shame that this beauty should not be seen and appreciated by others. Every crystal was a masterpiece of design and no one design was ever repeated. When a snowflake melted, that design was forever lost. Just that much beauty was gone, without leaving any record behind."[1]

During his lifetime, he captured over five thousand images of crystals that, even at sub-zero temperatures, were ephemeral, passing quickly from solid to vapor (see figs. 5.1–5.6). In the last few years of the nineteenth century his work gained more public attention when he published an article stating that no two snowflakes are alike. With the heart of a poet, he described the inner beauty of each crystal, and with the mind of a scientist, wondered why the shapes and sizes varied so much from one storm to the next. It was his scientific bent that prompted him to keep detailed meteorological records on the snowflakes and earned him the first, albeit modest, research grant ever given by the American Meteorological Society in 1924.

"A careful study of this internal structure not only reveals new and far greater elegance of form than the simple outlines exhibit, but by means of these wonderfully delicate and exquisite figures much may be learned of the history of each crystal, and the changes through which it has passed in its journey through cloudland. Was ever life history written in more dainty hieroglyphics!"[2]

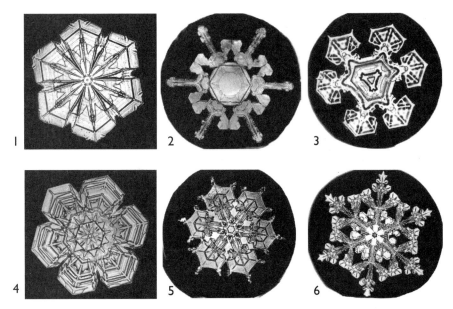

Figs. 5.1–5.6. Examples of Wilson Bentley's six-sided snowflakes.
Photos: Wilson Bentley Digital Archives of the Jericho Historical Society/
snowflakebentley.com.

Referring to the figures above, we can see that while each crystal has a unique formation, each one still has six rays in common. These crystals bear a striking resemblance to the water crystals photographed by Dr. Masaru Emoto.

THE WONDER OF WATER

Dr. Masaru Emoto was born July 22, 1943, in Yokohama, Japan. A graduate of Yokohama Municipal University (Department of Humanities and Sciences), with emphasis in international studies, he also obtained a Doctor of Alternative Medicine in 1992 from the Open International University. Shortly after, he was introduced to the concept of micro cluster water and Magnetic Resonance Analysis technology, thus beginning his fascination with water.

He authored several bestselling books, including *Messages from Water* and *The Hidden Messages in Water,* which contain photographs

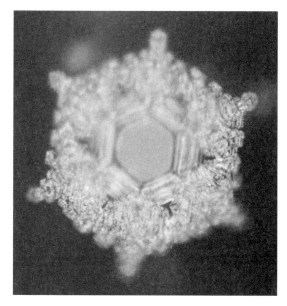

Fig. 5.7. Dr. Emoto's water crystal image with positive energy.
Copyright, Office Masaru Emoto, LLC.

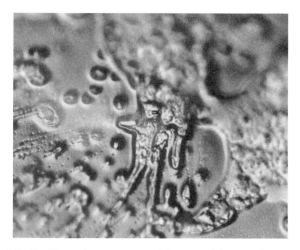

Fig. 5.8. Dr. Emoto's water crystal image with negative energy.
Copyright, Office Masaru Emoto, LLC.

of ice crystals (as depicted in figs. 5.7 and 5.8) and how they change in response to surrounding energy and vibration. His ideas were also included in the movie *What the Bleep Do We Know?*

What his pictures reveal is that when water is exposed to positive thoughts, beautiful music (usually classical), or reverence in the form of prayer or meditation, the crystals formed beautiful symmetrical crystals (see fig. 5.7). When exposed to negative thoughts such as hatred, criticism, ridicule, or chaotic music such as heavy metal, the water took on ugly shapes that lacked organization, symmetry, and balance, instead appearing with a deformed shape (see fig. 5.8). Dr. Emoto's goal was to unite the world in understanding that consciously emanating positivity contributes to healing, not only of Earth's waters, but also the human body, composed as it is of 70 percent water.

Mainstream science defines his life's work as pseudoscience and in response he joked once in an interview about our "double-blind" experiments living up to their name. When a methodology expects to see results that are exactly alike every single time, it fails to recognize the infinite expression of nature in response to life. The geometric formations of the snowflakes and water crystals reveal to us that, while patterns do repeat in nature, nature itself offers infinite ways to express creative change and cannot be forced into sameness.

COVALENT BONDING AND WATER "MEMORY"

To the matter of whether or not water crystals actually change when exposed to different states of human consciousness, music, and words, two-time Nobel Prize-winner Linus Pauling (1901–1994) was the first to introduce the theory of water memory transfer. Through a process known as covalent bonding, two atoms join together to form a molecule, and electrons "orbit" around the water molecule, much like planets around the sun. In unhealthy water, one of the electrons is missing, creating an opportunity for unhealthy microbes to gather.[3]

To explain covalent bonding, Pauling introduced two new concepts based on quantum mechanics: bond-orbital hybridization and bond resonance. "Hybridization reorganizes an atom's electron cloud so that some electrons assume positions favorable for bonding. Since the carbon atom can form four bonds, tetrahedrally arranged—a central structural feature of organic chemistry . . . Resonance is a rapid jumping of electrons back and forth between two or more possible positions in a bond network. Resonance makes a major contribution to the structural geometry and stability of many substances . . . for which a static, non-resonating bond system would be inadequate."[4]

In the last edition of his publication "The Nature of the Chemical Bond," Pauling said: "We may ask what the next step in the search for an understanding of the nature of life will be. I think that it will be the elucidation of the nature of the electromagnetic phenomena involved in mental activity in relation to the molecular structure of brain tissue. I believe that thinking, both conscious and unconscious, and short-term memory involves electromagnetic phenomena in the brain, interacting with the molecular (material) patterns of long-term memory, obtained from inheritance or experience."[5]

Modern brain science continues to gather evidence that neurons and glial cells, particularly the aquaporin-4 abundantly present in glial cells, play an essential role in brain function, thereby accentuating the functional role of water molecules in the brain.[6] If Pauling is correct that the state of water molecules affects brain function, and resonance affects the formation of water molecules, Dr. Emoto's work involving the impact of vibration on water crystals is certainly worthy of scientific consideration.

THE SIGNIFICANCE OF SIX

Emoto and Bentley were not the first to wonder about the formation of water crystals, specifically the significance of the hexagonal shape. Johannes Kepler, astronomer, astrologer, and mathematician, best known for his laws of planetary motion, also published a book titled *The Six-Cornered Snowflake: A New Year's Gift* in 1611.

As Kepler walked home one evening, contemplating what sort of gift would suit a friend whom he described as "a lover of nothing," it began to snow. Remembering that the Latin word for snowflake is *nix,* he concluded he had found the perfect gift: " . . . and a few scattered flakes fell on my coat, all six-cornered, with tufted radii . . . Here indeed was a most desirable New Year's gift . . . one worthy as well of a mathematician . . . since it descends from the sky and bears a likeness to the stars." In the book he explains " . . . when it begins to snow . . . the first particles . . . adopt the shape of small, six-cornered stars, there must be a particular cause; for if it happened by chance, why would they always fall with six corners, and not with five, or seven, as long as they are still scattered and distinct, and before they are driven into a confused mass?"[7]

Kepler never found the answer to the snowflake hexagon, instead focusing on planetary phenomena. However, we will explore the link between his planetary discoveries and the six-cornered snowflake that fascinated him shortly. For now our focus will remain on a simpler explanation for the formation of water crystals. Water molecules contain crystalline lattices that have a sixfold symmetry resembling that of the honeycomb (see fig. 5.9). The formation they take depends upon processes called *faceting* and *branching*. Faceting creates simpler structures and branching more complex ones. The influences of temperature and humidity determine which of the processes becomes more dominant, resulting in the many diverse snow crystal formations.[8]

Bentley believed that the forces producing hexagonal rings were electromagnetic and in 1910, proposed an electromagnetic water model, years before Linus Pauling discussed electromagnetic energy and molecular structure.[9]

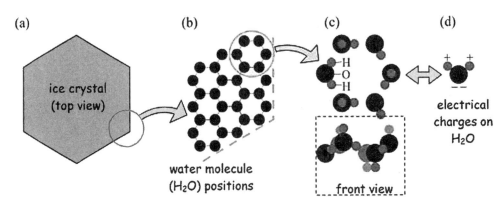

Fig. 5.9. Stages of the ice crystal hexagonal formation.
Copyright Jon Nelson, Redmond Physical Sciences.

HEXAGONAL RELATIONSHIP TO ELEMENTS

In chapter 2, we briefly looked at the math and music of Pythagoras, including the five geometric shapes that correspond to fire, earth, air, water, and ether (universe, quintessence). We will resume our discussion of Pythagorean concepts in chapter 7. First put forth by Plato, these five geometric forms were described as the fundamental building blocks of the universe. Today, scientist and director of research at the Resonance Project Foundation (RPF), Nassim Haramein upholds this theory.

Haramein contends that the platonic solids can be applied to understanding the geometry inherent in space-time and the vacuum of space as "an infinite tetrahedral array that creates the holofractographic structure of space-time on all scales which gives rise to everything we call 'ordinary matter.'"[10] This tetrahedral array is linked to what Buckminster Fuller called the Vector Equilibrium (VE), discussed a little later.

While certain shapes connect to others, only the hexagon corresponds to the symmetries of all five platonic solids (see figs. 5.10 and 5.11). Since nature uses the most efficient means available to create structure, we see hexagons repeatedly in examples such as the center of a carrot slice or the top of a tomato or green pepper. Another example that may be observed is watching the froth of bubbles settle into a hexagonal pattern, six-around-one, as they seek stability and rest.[11]

When it comes to more elaborate structuring, nature uses the

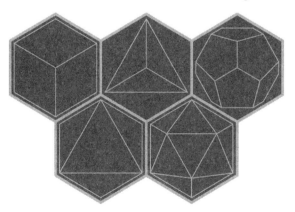

Fig. 5.10. Hexagonal frame of five platonic solids.
Courtesy of Graham Steele, www.hexnet.org.

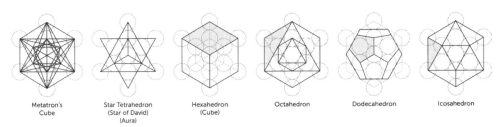

| Metatron's Cube | Star Tetrahedron (Star of David) (Aura) | Hexahedron (Cube) | Octahedron | Dodecahedron | Icosahedron |

Fig. 5.11. Fruit of Life (also Flower of Life) pattern shown in platonic solids. Illustrated by MidnightLightning (CC BY-SA 3.0).

hexagon through a process called tessellation, or "packaging."[12] explains that when circles tessellate they create curved triangular gaps; however, when converted to hexagons, there is equality in every direction, as with the honeycomb in figure 5.9b.

HEXAGONS IN OUTER SPACE

Strange as it may seem, and in accordance with the mirroring of the expression "As above, so below," hexagons occur in outer space as well. In 1980 and 1981 the Voyager expeditions photographed a hexagonal vortex on Saturn's north pole; later, clearer photos were available when NASA's Cassini mission captured images of the hexagon (fig. 5.12). In keeping with the context of the macrocosm, what's amazing is that each side of Saturn's hexagon exceeds the Earth's diameter!

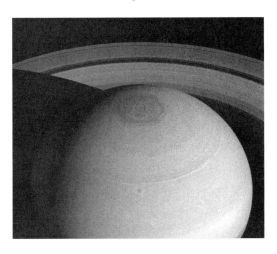

Fig. 5.12. Hexagon on Saturn's north pole. "PIA18274-Saturn-NorthPolarHexagon-Cassini-20140402" by NASA/JPL-Caltech/ Space Science Institute, www.nasa.gov/sites/default /files/pia18274_full.jpg.

Haramein posits that the hexagon is a fundamental geometric structure in the universe, formed by the tetrahedral structure (basic to chemical bonds as stated by Pauling), bonding together in a perfectly balanced state, which is both hexagonal and tetrahedral in nature.[13] RPF staff member Marshall Lefferts explains

To understand this concept of a geometry of perfect equilibrium, we looked to the pioneering work of Buckminster Fuller who first discerned this geometry in 1917 and came to call it the Vector Equilibrium in 1940. As a geometric form it is known as a cuboctahedron, but as an expression of ultimate equilibrium he gave it this name to describe its energetic condition—vectors that are all the same in length to the center and around the circumference. The VE, as it's also called, is the only geometry that satisfies this condition (others, such as the platonic forms, have equal-length edges, but shorter or longer vectors to their center point).[14]

In perfect balance, the Vector Equilibrium represents a state wherein all fluctuation and change cease. It is analogous to a vacuum of space (black hole), zero point, or unified field. Fuller described it this way: "The vector equilibrium is the zero starting point for all happenings or nonhappenings; it is the empty theater and empty circus and empty Universe, ready to accommodate any act and any audience."[15]

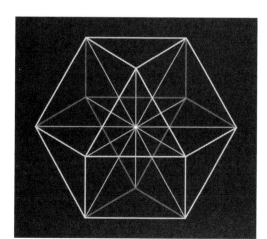

Fig. 5.13. Regular Vector Equilibrium. Source: Marshall Lefferts, www.cosmometry.net.

In order for anything to manifest either physically or metaphysically in an observable/measurable way, there must be fluctuation in the unified field. According to contemporary physics, before any fluctuation occurs, this unified field exists as pure potential and contains an infinite amount of energy. From the spiritual perspective, it also contains infinite creative (and consciousness) potential.[16]

At the center point of the Vector Equilibrium an array of equal vectors can be extended into infinity producing what is known as the Isotropic Vector Matrix (IVM). "Isotropic means 'all the same,' Vector means 'line of energy,' and Matrix means 'a pattern of lines of energy.' It is this full isotropic vector matrix that can be seen as the infinitely-present-at-all-scales-and-in-perfect-equilibrium geometry of the zero-point Unified Field. Every point in this matrix is a potential center point of a VE around which a condition of dynamic fluctuation may arise to manifest."[17]

It's also possible to create the geometry of the Vector Equilibrium using thirteen spheres of the same diameter (see fig. 5.14). With one sphere at the center, acting as "nucleus" and twelve spheres surrounding it, the

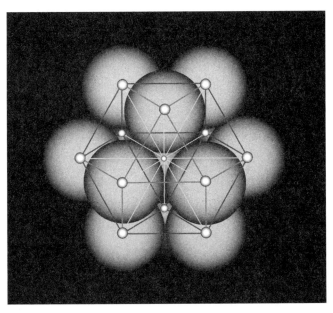

Fig. 5.14. Spherical Vector Equilibrium. (Note the tiny spheres that add up to thirteen when combined with larger spheres.) Source: Marshall Lefferts, www.cosmometry.net.

center of each sphere then becomes its own center point. The lines connecting their centers become the vectors of Vector Equilibrium. In geometry, this twelve-around-one system is analogous to the twelve-tone music scale, the twelve signs of the zodiac, and the twelve apostles of Christ.[18]

REFERENCES TO ANCIENT ZODIACS

The twelve-around-one theme can be found everywhere in ancient culture. According to author Michael Schneider, "prehistoric" civilizations as far back as 12,000 BCE left signs of mathematic sophistication, modeling their communities on the pattern of the twelve constellations, and dividing their land into twelve regions accordingly. One example he cited was ancient Ireland, with Tara—the location of the High King's celestial court—at the center, and the outlying regions designed to mirror the zodiac.[19] The significance of this as it relates to "six" is that, in the zodiac circle, there are always six constellations above the horizon and six constellations below the horizon, with Earth at the center (in the geodesic perspective).

Another ancient phenomenon related to spherical Vector Equilibrium is the Fruit of Life or Flower of Life pattern. Looking back at Figure 5.11 you will see the preliminary stage of the Flower of Life (FOL) pattern framing each platonic solid; figure 5.15 shows FOL in its

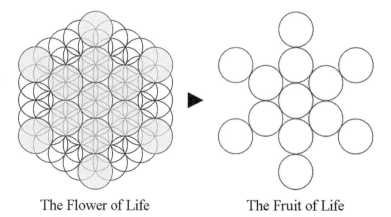

The Flower of Life   The Fruit of Life

Fig. 5.15. Flower of Life/Fruit of Life pattern.
Illustrated by MidnightLightning (CC BY-SA 3.0).

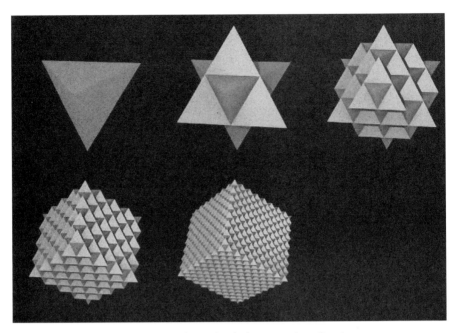

Fig. 5.16. Fractal tetrahedral stage of replication.
Copyright Resonance Academy and Nassim Haramein.

typical form when more spheres are added that connect from the central sphere and from the center of each additional sphere. This symbol is found in sacred temples all over the world, and has a connection to the I Ching, which we will explore a little later.

Because of its perfect symmetry, the Vector Equilibrium allows continuous replication inwardly and outwardly. Mathematics describes this as fractal tetrahedral wherein new vectors are created unceasingly to maintain equilibrium throughout a particular system, such as the universe. The importance of the repeating vectors toward the infinitesimally small as well as the infinitely large, maintaining equilibrium with harmonic intervals, cannot be overstated. (In fig. 5.16 we see the fractal tetrahedral image as it replicates from one cell to multiple cells.) The interval is what defines all torus systems that organize matter and create natural dimensions of the vacuum that follow the golden ratio (Phi and the Flower of Life) found everywhere in nature.[20]

EMPTY SPACE "MATTERS"

If we operate on the supposition that the hexagon is the fundamental geometric structure in the fabric of space-time, we need to look at what exactly makes up "space." Our world is comprised of more space than matter, but as humans we tend to place a higher priority on all the "solid stuff." (And that often makes us dense!) Physics tells us that space makes up 99.99999 percent of all reality. But is space really empty? As with any new field of exploration, controversy exists, and in this case the two physics theories that do not agree are general relativity and quantum theory.

One new theory that I offer here comes from Haramein's research, which is carried out through the Resonance Project Foundation, and is offered as public classes and discussions in an online forum through the Resonance Academy. On the topic of space, he explains that in modern physics we think of the universe as being comprised of atoms, and those atoms bond together forming molecules, which in turn make up all matter. A basic hydrogen atom has at its center a single proton, the volume of which is thought to be 2.5×10^{-39} cm^3 (10^{-45} m^3). He continues to explain that, since electrons are considered to be point particles that have no volume, "we can simply divide the volume of the proton to find out just how full the hydrogen atom actually is . . ."

The following information is taken from The Resonance Academy Module 4, Section 2, "Unified Physics," and edited by The Resonance Project research team for this publication:

$$(2.5 \times 10^{-39} \text{ cm}^3 \, / \, 6.2 \times 10^{-25} \text{ cm}^3) \times 100$$
$$(4 \times 10^{-15}) \times 100$$
$$4 \times 10^{-13} \text{ percent}$$
$$\text{Percent Full} = 0.0000000000004 \text{ percent}$$

Using the "standard logic of particle physics," his calculations result in the hydrogen atom being 99.9999 percent empty space . . . !

However, he goes on to explain that the reason things do not simply "pass through" other things (particles) is because empty space is actually not empty. Vacuums, according to Haramein, are full of energy, and atoms and electrons are actually electromagnetic fields: "In the case of the atom, electrons are not simply points in space, they are fields. Even the radius of the proton is described as the 'charge radius' of the proton because all that can be identified as a proton is a charge density in a region of space, or a field, that we call a particle."

Haramein's research also looks at the construction of black holes, and considers the connected universe as one Black Whole.[21] In his paper "The Schwarzschild Proton," Haramein calculated the density of vacuum energy contained within a proton volume and found it to be 10^{55}g/proton volume, which is equal to the mass-energy of the observable universe. This value is found from defining the Planck spherical unit and calculating the amount of Planck spherical units inside one proton. (Max Planck, 1858–1947, is known as the originator of quantum theory.)

Haramein stated that the volume of our universe (10^{55} g) is close to what is called the "critical limit," an amount of energy needed to push our universe to expand and accelerate. The critical limit is analogous to the amount of radiant energy, often called dark energy, which is required to expand the universe at the rate we currently observe. Haramein also points out that the mass-energy of the observable universe, $\sim 10^{55}$ grams, with a radius of 10^{28} cm happens to obey the Schwarzschild condition of black holes.[22] Even more interesting is that everything has at its center a point of singularity and stillness, a black hole: "The proton, the sun and the galaxy are all centered by various scale black holes, all centered by singularity. Everything in the universe is centered by stillness. Space-time curls like water going down the drain to the singularity in the center of black holes on all scales in the infinite scalar . . . fabric of the vacuum . . . "[23]

HOLOGRAPHIC ENCODING

Haramein's quantized solution to gravity encompasses a theory called *holographic encoding* whereby the information of all protons is recorded inside every individual proton. Supposing this is true, it certainly fits with ancient theories regarding the microcosm-macrocosm connection.

Beginning with the premise that the mass-energy value of all of the protons in the universe ($\sim 10^{55}$ grams) is present inside each single proton, Haramein explains that it is analogous to music on a hard drive. This music fits into a tiny region of magnetic media, and while the actual musicians are not found in that space, the music they record is present.

However, the difference lies in the fact that it is not a "one and done" recording. The media, in theory, would actually be connected to the musicians on a continuous basis so that, as with a computer network, the information is being updated constantly. "Just like the media of a hard drive, where the information is embedded in the magnetic medium electromagnetically, the electromagnetic structure of the quantum vacuum energy holographically encodes information at the Planck bit scale inside of each proton, what we can call 'spacememory.' Just like the interference pattern that records the image information on a holographic plate, all the information of all other protons is holographically recorded inside each and every individual proton."[24]

This analogy fits well with the Pythagorean concept of the universe as the music of the spheres, which we will address in chapter 7.

As previously stated, Haramein's unified physics is on the cutting edge and is accompanied by much debate. For our purposes, it is relevant to ponder the implications of such interaction between electromagnetic fields and magnetic "recordings," particularly as we continue to consider planetary effects on human life.

THE HARMONIC UNIVERSE

Johannes Kepler once said: "Where there is matter, there is geometry." Perhaps a revision better suited to our discussion would be "Where there is mass, there is geometry." If empty space is not truly empty, holding instead a massive amount of density, it stands to reason that within it is the geometry of which Kepler spoke. His work was built upon Pythagorean principles, including the platonic (or perfect) solids discussed above and their correspondence to the five elements.

Born in sixteenth-century Germany during a time when religious conflicts arose between the Roman Catholics and Lutherans, Kepler, who was also a theologian, searched for answers that would prove the world was created in harmony. He believed that that the heavenly bodies did influence human life, but also felt that certain astrological predictions were inclined to manipulate influential people. Where astronomy was concerned, he questioned Aristotelian views in support of Copernican's heliocentrism at a time when such exploration risked embarrassment. "The idea that taking another look at the basic assumptions of astronomy could be beneficial, even necessary, did not occur to the vast majority of philosophers."[25]

With regard to nature, Kepler understood it within the context of mass, size, and quantity. He believed that the mind of God was mathematical, and that space was structured accordingly. "The more we think in numbers . . . the clearer our thinking becomes."[26] Many questions concerned him, such as what determined the distance between the planets, why were the orbits a specific size, and what do those measurements mean?

While teaching a class one day, he drew an equilateral triangle contained within a circle, and inspiration struck. He drew another circle inside the triangle and realized that the ratio of the larger to the smaller circle corresponded to the ratio of the orbits of Saturn to Jupiter. In that moment, he had begun his discovery that geometric figures determine the space between the planetary orbits. He began to experiment with other geometric figures, plugging them into the known planetary orbits, looking for a pattern. At first this failed because he was using two-dimensional shapes. When it dawned on him that space was three-dimensional, he began to use the platonic solids and that's when things began to make more sense.

In 1596, he published *Mysterium Cosmographicum,* the first astronomical work that supported Copernican theory. Although the publication was groundbreaking, it still contained errors that launched further exploration, specifically regarding the planetary orbits.[27] But by the time he had completed the work, Kepler was more convinced than ever that science and religion were part of one system, and he set about proving their congruency. In 1609 he published the first two laws of planetary motion, followed by the third law in 1619.

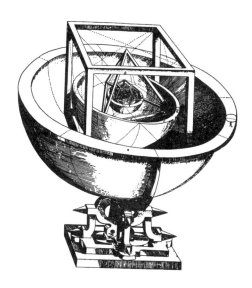

Fig. 5.17. Kepler's platonic solid model of the solar system from *Mysterium Cosmographicum* (1596).

LAWS OF PLANETARY MOTION

Danish astronomer Tycho Brahe had supported Kepler's research; before Brahe's death in 1601, he set Kepler to the task of figuring out Mars's orbit. It was this endeavor that lead to the first law of planetary motion. Kepler wanted to know the radius of Mars's orbit, where its speed varied, and by how much. It took an exhaustive nine hundred pages of calculations (now performed with calculus that was not available then) before he arrived at a numerical value representing the orbit of Mars. But it still did not solve the issue, and it wasn't until he accidentally "discovered" the second law of equal areas that he could define the first law of elliptical motion (see fig. 5.18). "The second law geometrically confirms that planets do not move at uniform speeds. Because equal areas are 'swept out' in equal time, the farther it is from the Sun, the less distance a planet must travel in the same time interval."[28]

The first law states that planets move in an elliptical motion around the sun, moving faster as they get closer to its gravitational force field. The second law explains that when measuring planetary movement within a specific period of time, no matter where that planet is in its orbit, there is an equal area carved out between the first distance covered (x) and the next distance (y), as depicted in figure 5.18.

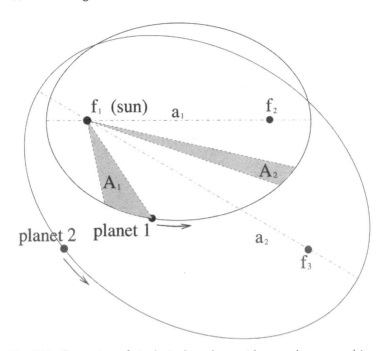

Fig. 5.18. Illustration of Kepler's three laws with two planetary orbits.
(1) The orbits are ellipses, with focal points f_1 and f_2 for the first planet
and f_1 and f_3 for the second planet. The Sun is placed in focal point f_1.
(2) The two shaded sectors A_1 and A_2 have the same surface area and the time
for planet 1 to cover segment A_1 is equal to the time to cover segment A_2.
(3) The total orbit times for planet 1 and planet 2 have a ratio $a_1^{3/2} : a_2^{3/2}$.
Illustration by Hankwang (CC BY-SA 3.0).

Throughout his life, Kepler would fight bouts of depression by returning to his work, tirelessly striving to prove that the world was structured in harmony. In 1617, turning his attention back to *Mysterium Cosmographicum,* fresh insights enabled him to put together the third law and most cherished work, *The Harmony of the World.* In the first two laws, he was comparing movement between the sun and a planet, between the central focal point and the orbiting object. In the third law, he was comparing the relationship between two objects that orbit the same body, for instance, between two planets orbiting the sun. (Please see fig. 5.18 for a mathematical description of the third law.)

In *Mysterium Cosmographicum,* the five solids are three-dimensional shapes that can be inscribed inside a sphere. In *The Harmony of the World* he divides them into three primary and two secondary figures. The three primaries are the cube, tetrahedron and dodecahedron, with the cube and dodecahedron also considered "male." The two secondary solids are the icosahedron and octahedron, considered female. The tetrahedron, while it is classified as primary, is neither male nor female; rather it is considered "hermaphrodite" because it is inscribed in itself.[29]

This I find interesting since it is the fractal tetrahedral that is believed to provide equilibrium within the Isotropic Vector Matrix. Furthermore, Kepler's cosmology describes the sphere (three-dimensional) as representing the Holy Trinity, and the two-dimensional plane representing the material world. He categorizes "knowable" shapes as those two-dimensional forms that can be constructed by a compass and a ruler, and "unknowable" shapes as those unable to be drawn in that manner.

> He then searched for combinations of the perfect solids and two-dimensional shapes that created ratios corresponding to musical harmony. These ratios would be physical expressions of the harmonious relationship between God and his creation, and the corresponding geometric shapes would become the building blocks of the universe . . . Further calculations convinced him that he had uncovered a multi-level system of planetary harmony that applied to the planets both individually and as a group. Soon he was describing the known planets as a choir, with each planet having a voice. "The heavenly motions are nothing but a continuous song for several voices (perceived by the intellect, not by the ear)."[30]

In the midst of this discovery, he uncovered an important ratio: the square of the orbital period is proportional to the cube of the mean distance from the sun. His third law of planetary motion had, for the first time, established a correlation between the orbital period and distance, thereby combining time and space in a single mathematical formula.[31]

THE MEDICINE CONNECTION

Kepler acknowledged that he was living in an exciting time when the convergence of brilliant minds was bringing back Hermetic principles, Paracelsian medicine, ancient alchemy, and the link between astronomy and medicine.

> After the birth of printing books became widespread. Hence everyone throughout Europe devoted himself to the study of literature . . . Every year, especially since 1563, the number of writings published in every field is greater than all those produced in the past thousand years. Through them there has today been created a new theology and a new jurisprudence; the Paracelsians have created medicine anew and the Copernicans have created astronomy anew. I really believe that at last the world is alive, indeed seething, and that the stimuli of these remarkable conjunctions did not act in vain.[32]

Today his words could easily apply, as it seems that now is a time when many of these ancient philosophies are rising to the surface again. If all planets, stars, and galaxies are torus energy systems defined by their central black hole (see fig. 5.19), and those black holes are points of singularity (zero point or stillness), how does that affect our creative capacity to heal? Recall Fuller's definition of the black hole (unified field) as being a place where infinite potential lies waiting to "accommodate any act or audience."

The paradox we face is that there is simultaneously a double torus spin, represented by the opposites yin and yang and circulating around the black hole of stillness where all potential lies in wait. When we lose our center, that zero point of gravity, we can spin out of control very easily. When we maintain balance and equilibrium, as the masters learned how to do in meditation, we stay grounded in a place of pure potentiality. This is the very definition of the Tao.

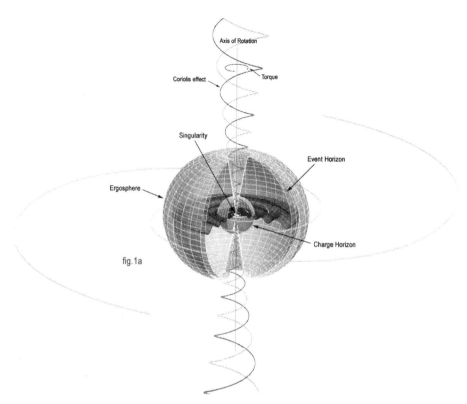

Fig. 5.19. Double torus at Earth's poles.
Copyright Resonance Academy and Nassim Haramein.

ENTER THE I CHING

The same double torus that occurs in planets, stars, and galaxies also occurs in the human anatomy (see fig. 5.21). But first we will examine the connection between the geometry of space and the I Ching. In a 2013 interview presented by Evolution TV, Haramein explains that the I Ching system, with its sixty-four hexagrams, can create a star tetrahedron that forms "the Flower of Life" (also known as the Fruit of Life and Merkaba).

The I Ching is comprised of six solid (yang) lines and six broken (yin) lines. Haramein noticed that the only three-dimensional geometry that the six solid yang lines can make is a tetrahedron. To make a star tetrahedron, the broken yin lines must be added so that they can pass

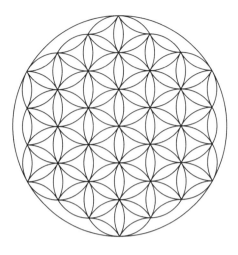

Fig. 5.20. Spherical tetrahedron forming the Flower of Life.

through the lines of the first tetrahedron, connecting the yang lines. When the star tetrahedron is created spherically, the Flower of Life is created.

Haramein is not alone in making this connection to the I Ching. In *The Secret of the Golden Flower,* Richard Wilhelm explains that the I Ching, alchemy, Flower of Life (or golden flower), and the golden mean are all part of the same system handed down in secret to protect the teachings during volatile periods throughout history. With regard to the I Ching, he explains: "The eight basic trigrams (Pa Kua) of the I Ching are . . . symbols for certain inner processes . . . "[33]

Wilhelm discusses the parallels between the teachings of Christ and those of the Tao. The Book of John says "'I baptize you with water: after me shall come one who will baptize with the Holy Ghost and with fire'; or: 'Except a man be born of water and of the spirit, he cannot enter into the kingdom of God.'"[34] It is understood, then, that the "kingdom of God" is the Tao, the elixir of life or, for the purpose of our discussion, the unified field, zero point, and singularity. "The Tao, then, the Way, governs man just as it does invisible and visible nature (heaven and earth) . . . The fundamental idea is that the Tao, though itself motionless, is the means of all movement and gives it law. Heavenly paths are those along which the constellations move; the path of man is the way along which he must travel." In another passage he explains: "A man who holds to the way of conservation all through life may reach the stage of the Golden Flower, which then frees the ego from the conflict of the opposites, and it again becomes part of the Tao, the undivided, great One."[35]

Despite the illusion of separation based upon the opposites, especially that of Eastern and Western traditions, the Tao and the unified field provide the "inner way" back to connection. By proxy, this examination of inner space affects the physical anatomy every bit as much as it does the soul.

IT'S IN OUR DNA

When we examine our DNA structure, we find that it displays both a "5" (penta) and a "6" (hexa) pattern in its molecular arrangement. The golden rectangle that joins the penta-hexa geometries is the double hydrogen bond in the phi ratio.[36]

According to researcher Steve Krakowski, the sixty-four hexagrams of the I Ching correspond to the sixty-four codons in the universal genetic code. The hexagrams are three symbols (combinations) of yin and yang (broken or unbroken) lines. The codons are composed of four

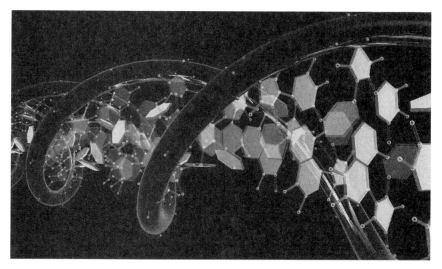

Fig. 5.21. DNA showing penta-hexa geometry.
Copyright Resonance Academy and Nassim Haramein.

nucleic acids taken three at a time. Krakowski set about determining which of the nucleic acids correspond to which I Ching symbol.[37]

He explains that the basic structure of the pyrimidine nucleic acids has six atoms and that of the purine nucleic acids has nine. Since "Old Yang" (two unbroken lines) corresponds to the number 9, and "Old Yin" (two broken lines) corresponds to the number 6, yang symbols were assigned to the purines, and the yin symbols to the pyrimidines. He then determined which yang symbol (old or young) would correspond to which purine nucleic acid (adenine or guanine).

Since energy is associated with yang, matter is associated with yin, and energy for bio-chemical processes in cells is provided by adenosine triphosphate, he correlated adenine with Old Yang. From this assignment, it followed that Old Yin (complement to Old Yang) would be assigned adenine's opposite—thymine. Lastly, Young Yang, assigned to guanine because it is a purine nucleic acid, its opposite, cytosine, he assigned to Young Yin.[38]

Whether Krakowski's speculations prove true or false, I find it a fascinating theory to consider given the nature of opposites and the function of yin and yang in anatomy.

AN-ATOM-Y AND GEOMETRY

Since we began our discussion with the microscopic forms found in water crystals, it seems fitting to end by taking a look at the human cell. An indicator that technological progress can be a friend to and, in all ways, support spiritual connection, is a recent discovery regarding the hexagonal shape of an atom.

In 2009, an IBM team from Zürich published their findings in the journal *Science,* showing images they captured of single molecules with exquisite detail; so detailed that the type of atomic bonds between their atoms could be discerned. As it happens, the same hexagonal shape found on Saturn in snowflakes and in ice crystals is also found in the image of the molecule.

"These new images will allow scientists to study . . . where electrons go during chemical reactions . . . they used a variant of a technique

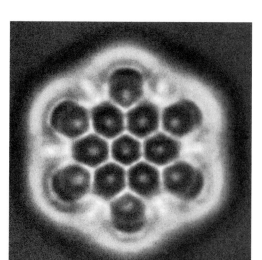

Fig. 5.22. The twelve-around-one hexagonal geometry of a human cell. © IBM Research/Science Source.

called atomic force microscopy (AFM). AFM uses a tiny metal tip that passes over a surface, where even tinier deflections are measured as the tip is scanned as it moves to and fro over a sample . . . The images showcased how long the atomic bonds are. The bright and dark spots correspond to higher and lower densities of electrons. There are different physical properties of different bonds."[39]

It seems that we have little to fear and much to gain from exploring the mathematical, mystical, and musical implications of the hexagon phenomenon in our world. To the ancients, the number 6 was analogous to time (duration, or chronology, derived from Chronos; and Saturn the sixth planet), and balance where both physical health and the environment are concerned because it holds the polarities in harmony. The equilibrium comes from recognizing the need for balance between the opposites. The equilibrium attained by this harmony of opposites also facilitates mastery of the Kundalini life force energy, which for the ancient alchemists, was the key to longevity and healing.

In the I Ching there are three unbroken yang lines and three broken yin lines; together there is perfect balance. Likewise in the body there are six yang and yin meridians. The number 6 represents harmony and soul in the hexad, which is formed by the union of two triangles representing masculine and feminine.[40] In Chinese medicine there are six yang and six yin meridians running energy through the body. Three yin and three yang meridians travel the upper body; three yin and three yang meridians travel the lower body. Maintaining a steady and balanced flow of energy along these meridians enables the body's internal organs to function optimally, thus supporting longevity.

In astrology, Saturn, which is the sixth planet from the sun, represents time, (Chronos/chronology) and governs the structure of things in the material realm. By coincidence or design, the sixth planet also has a hexagon on its north pole. The sixth house governs physical health, life's daily routine and details in the physical world. Its sign, Virgo, is a *mutable* earth sign (refer to chapter 4), requiring minute fluctuation and adjustment in order to maintain optimal health. Its opposite is Pisces (water), representing the nebulous sea of emotion and subtle spirituality. To the alchemists, immortality was achieved by removing the subtle (Pisces) from the material (Virgo), ascending to the world of spirit, and then returning to the body reborn.

Regardless of the name we choose to identify the process (Tao, the Way, unified field, zero point, stillness, or savior), the process is experienced in the same way. The path to health, longevity, and inner peace is achieved not by removing the opposite or opposites, but by reconciling them and maintaining equilibrium amid eternal change.

6

COSMIC LIGHT IN INNER AND OUTER SPACE

Having considered some of the correspondences between the infinitesimal and monumental forms in our universe, we will now consider matters of human anatomy, the role of ancient language, and astrology more closely. In keeping our focus on a particular element, this discussion will look at fire. It was the most sacred element to the ancients due to its association with spiritual light as well as being a source of life, energy, and generative power. The nature of light in all its forms is essential to understanding our individual responsibility for our health and our role on this planet.

Continuing with the Hermetic concept "As above, so below" and the reconciliation of opposites, it's important to keep in mind the relationship between darkness ("empty" space) and light, like that of yin with yang, and how one fuels the other. Put another way, light penetrates the darkness. Masculine energy seeds the feminine womb space, thereby creating life.

According to the ancients, both the planetary bodies of Earth and the human anatomy contain portals of energy where it is said immortals can commune with mortals, where the energy of light is carried into, and facilitated by, the darkness, like yin and yang (chapter 3). They also understood that the planets in our solar system influence life on Earth, providing the means for humans, specifically initiates trained in the sacred rituals, to access higher dimensions through the activation of cosmic light.

Author Vashist Vaid states that the Akashic field—known as

Arupa in India (unmanifested realm) to the Rupa (manifested realm)—includes, in order of magnitude: galaxies, constellations, solar systems, and planets. This universal electricity expresses itself according to the universal law of the "will to do good." According to Vaid, electromagnetism is created by the two principles of darkness and light, divine mother and divine father, which give birth to the balancing principle known as the "son aspect" or solar fire.[1]

The biblical quote "There is nothing new under the sun" (Ecclesiastes 1:9, NASB) becomes a guiding motif as we explore recent discoveries that ancient anatomists are likely to have understood.

THE MYSTERY OF MELANIN

It's important to keep in mind that the priests of the ancient world viewed the body as an intelligent organism divinely designed to access higher consciousness, as discussed in previous chapters when addressing inner alchemy and the management of Kundalini life force. In *Dark Light Consciousness,* Edward Bruce Bynum, Ph.D., clinical psychologist and director of behavioral medicine at University of Massachusetts at Amherst, traced an evolution of the human brain whereby he describes that dark matter on the surface of the brain increased its capacity to absorb light. "We see that over time there is a gradual increase in its [the brain's] capacity to absorb light. This is because there is an increasing darkness that covers its surface. This darkness gives it the capacity to absorb light."[2]

He describes the brain's threefold structure, which includes the reptilian brain stem, the midbrain of the limbic system, and the highly, albeit not completely, developed neocortex (new brain). The evolutionary phenomenon in the brain is quite complex, and seems to have something to do with the presence of neuromelanin (melanin in the brain), and its ability to "fold space" as Bynum puts it. Melanin, not to be confused with melatonin, is produced by cells called melanocytes, which provide pigmentation to skin, eyes, and hair. Melatonin, on the other hand, is involved in the entrainment (synchronization) of the circadian rhythm of physiological functions including sleep, and it functions in such a way as to anticipate "the daily onset of darkness."

However, according to Bynum, what's interesting about the function of neuromelanin is that it creates a coiling effect reminiscent of the serpent so sacred to ancient anatomists.

> These three and a half turnings . . . parallel the three and a half coils of the shining serpent of the perennial traditions sleeping at the bottom end or tail of the spine. Their union and awakening is the marriage of science and spirit . . . Each surface of these three unfolding brain structures is infused with the dark living current of neuromelanin from the brain stem to the neocortex. The curling of planes is happening within the bounds of the skull and creates the template for the perception of inner space within space, of enfolding inward higher dimensions.[3]

Apparently neuromelanin is highly sensitive to subtle electromagnetic activity, including the ability to absorb light (including through the pineal gland or vestigial "third eye"), and believed to be the primary factor (in addition to the coiling effect) contributing to the

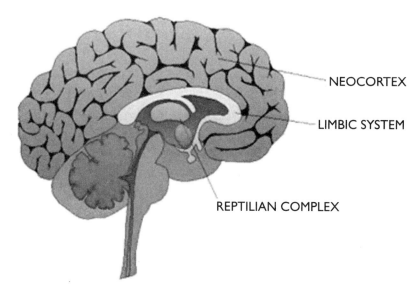

Fig. 6.1. Reptilian, limbic, and neocortex sections of the brain.
Image by Bruce Blaus (CC BY-SA 4.0).

brain's evolution. "In a process and structural sense, neuromelanin . . . is . . . involved in the brain's evolutionary folding and the perception of the unfolding of space. There is every reason to suspect that neuromelanin is implicated in the capacity of consciousness to fold space."[4]

Bynum addresses the difference between melanin of the skin, which has more to do with pigmentation, and neuromelanin in the brain, by explaining that neuromelanin "is a deep structure phenomenon" stemming from universal human experience with roots that transcend racial implications.[5]

However, melanin elsewhere in human anatomy does also reveal connections to the "serpentine spiral" and kundalini energy, as does the "anatomy" of Earth. Bynum explains that Earth itself has geodynamic forces that slowly spiral up into the terrestrial atmosphere and interact with the body's internal anatomy and central nervous system. The membrane surrounding each of the body's organs has the ability to absorb light and subtle electromagnetic energy related to the bioelectrical properties of melanin. Bynum states that this internal function constitutes the "matrix" with which the body is able to detect, absorb, and transduce geodynamic forces through the "light body" or energy field, which finds its physiologic root in melanin.

> Beyond the brain and brain stem, this melanin is represented in ample amounts in our internal organs . . . heart, lungs, kidneys, and gastro-intestinal (GI) tract, all contained in a structure bounded by skin. Melanin is able to . . . shift energy, from one state to another, from vibration to sound, to heat, to light. Since all forms of energy are related to each other it is not difficult to see that the subtle energy field of the body referred to in the esoteric traditions as . . . the energy body, the etheric body, the light or luminous body . . . is connected to an energy field that may partially be generated by the bioelectrical capacities of melanin in and on the surface of our inner organs is partially why we believe that the sensitive human nervous system can detect geodynamic forces arising from within the Earth.[6]

According to Bynum's experience, another interesting characteristic of melanin is that it has a tetrahedral shape. The significance of this shape speaks to our chemical and molecular structure as well as the platonic solid associated with the element of fire. The tetrahedral shape is the same as that of the pyramid.

> The tetrahedron is the only three-dimensional shape whose vertices are the same distance from each other. Apart from the sphere no other solids have fewer than 4 faces or 4 vertices. While the sphere encloses the most volume capable of holding all the solid shapes, space within the tetrahedron is minimal. This makes the tetrahedron the strongest and most stable solid as its root shape is the Triangle. Tetrahedrons are common in organic and inorganic chemistry. Many elementary molecules use it as a frame, for example . . . CH4 [methane], C2H6 [ethane] and amino acids. In each of these three molecules, a carbon of nitrogen atom sits at the centre of the tetrahedron at whose 4 corners reside 4 smaller hydrogen atoms.[7]

This geometric similarity to ancient structures at sacred sites is likely more than coincidence. It is also likely more than coincidence that the sacred sound "om" is shown to create the vibrational shape of a tetrahedron (see fig. 6.3).

We explore in greater detail the effects of sound on matter in chapter 8, but due to the tetrahedral connection to light, it is important to mention here that due to "the sound vibration 'om' in its physical manifestation . . . produces the image of the Sri Yantra . . . This is the classical Hindu image in which there are triangles within triangles within still other triangles. The four-dimensional sound of 'om' (length,

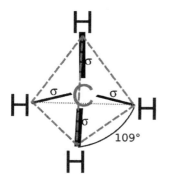

Fig. 6.2. Tetrahedral geometry of the carbon atom (CC BY-SA 3.0).

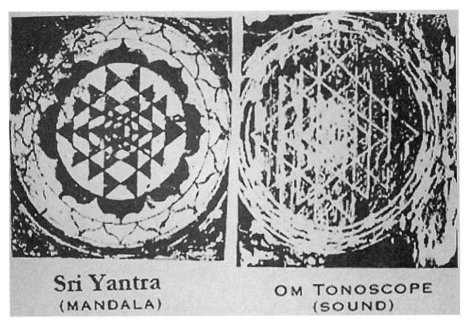

Fig. 6.3. Sri Yantra Mandala comparison to Ohm Tonoscope.

width, depth of physical space, and time or duration) vibrated through this instrument [tonoscope] will manifest as this particular physical figure in two dimensions . . . these triangles are also connected with the shape of the tetrahedron or pyramid shape."[8]

Bynum states that melanin as biochemical substrate has an intimate connection with the wave nature of light due to its interaction with electromagnetic energy. This is because "as a physical substrate of the human body it is also woven into the electromagnetic field, and can act as a gateway to higher dimensional forces."[9]

Author Manly Hall recounts Plato's description of the body as a sarcophagus of the soul, referring to that immortal potentiality held within its form that could only be freed by way of initiation or "death."[10] The ancients considered the two to be synonymous, just as Jesus Christ recapitulated: "Except a man be born again, he cannot see the kingdom of God." (John 3:3, King James Version). This teaching is important to keep in mind as we now go back to explore ancient Egyptian practices, particularly that of potential priests and their initiations.

THE NATURE OF LIGHT

Just as there are currents, waves, whirlpools, and cycles that exist in the body of water we call the ocean, it seems reasonable to consider that there are currents, waves, whirlpools (wormholes), and cycles in the light that permeate our inner and outer worlds. The phenomenal world is the objective and largely "known" world in which we witness light manifesting as objects in space. The non-phenomenal world is beyond the four dimensions we readily experience.

Yet access to a fifth-dimensional realm and beyond becomes possible when we consider some implications of melanin. Because of its ability to transduce the subtle electromagnetic field, it may behave as a bridge between the phenomenal and non-phenomenal dimensions. Therefore, the superluminal (also superconsciousness) realm becomes accessible through spiritual practice, meditation, dreams, and other disciplines. Another way to describe the phenomenal and non-phenomenal realms is through the terms *objective light* and *subjective light*. Bynum describes light (with both wave and particle functions) as an energetic force not restricted by time and space; rather it uses time and space as a means for manifestation.[11] Light propagated through the universe provides a window into past times dependent upon the place and moment in space wherein one intersects with it.

Quantum mechanics holds that the act of observation influences particle behavior upon that observation taking place (the famous Heisenberg uncertainty principle). Objective light in the form of radio, microwave, broadband, and laser can more easily be measured. However, when dealing with subjective light, because it involves individual consciousness, it is potentially infinite in its form(s) of manifestation, yet no less "real" to its observers.[12] "It is a misplaced ideal and perhaps delusion of contemporary science that in order to become objective and see clearly one has to abstract human consciousness from the equation itself. Implicit in the equations of relativity and to a growing extent quantum mechanics, is the irreducibility of the witness or 'observer,' which in our case is human consciousness."[13]

There is every reason to consider, therefore, that "death" is no longer the only experience by which human consciousness can experience higher dimensions. Both ancient texts and recent research suggests that this type of spiritual soul travel is real and was, in fact, part of the priests' initiation process.

The process also involves recognition of the correlation between the body's organs and the planetary bodies in our solar system. Before discussing the body's planetary temple it's important to understand the role that language played in our understanding of ancient texts describing cosmic phenomenon.

LANGUAGE OF THE LUMINARIES

In order to pass sacred knowledge on to trained initiates with the "eyes to see and ears to hear," language was laden with symbolism. The ancients used symbols in ways to commit certain things to memory. Without recognition of their original context, modern interpretation of certain words has come to mean something quite different from their original meanings. French occultist, student of sacred geometry, and Egyptologist R. A. Schwaller de Lubicz (1887–1961) pointed out that our language and definition of words has served to limit our understanding of the concepts upon which the ancients based their work. He suggested that our language, being built upon a conventional alphabet, creates mechanical ways of composing and understanding the meanings of certain words. "It may be said that the combinations of these letters are almost infinite: true, but the number of words is limited by notions already acquired. Thought can also examine observed phenomena and seek the causes . . . *but as soon as it approaches the metaphysical, it can no longer find in our languages and forms of writing the means of expressing itself.* Abstract ideas, formulated in words for which we lack the concepts, are objectified and lose their significance."[14] (Italics added.)

We find ancient texts were very likely based on astronomical observations having to do with the movement of light. Karl Anderson, author of *Astrology of the Old Testament or the Lost World Regained*, provided one such example.[15] Anderson writes that *Genesis* is derived from *Gen-Isis* (*Isis* being the Egyptian moon goddess). "In the beginning God said, 'Let there be light: and there was light.' Light first springs from the first point in which the sun ascends at daybreak, or the life of nature commences in the point Aries." He explains that when God says "Let us make man in our image," 'us' refers to the luminaries Osiris (sun) and Isis (moon)—the positive and negative principles, respectively. Osiris, as the sun, is the life giver, and Isis, as the moon, is the producer. One represents spirit (sun as the principle form of light), and the other, matter (moon as light reflected in the darkness). In Sanskrit the word *Maia* is equivalent to the Egyptian *Isis* (or *Mot/Maat*). The celestial virgin and Queen of Heaven is equivalent to the ancient Greek Ceres (the maternal aspect of the feminine, bread giver, manna producer). She brought the "harvest," producing life in its fullest expression, and thus was perceived as the heavenly provider. Because the harvest moon was lovelier than at any other moon cycle, it came to be described as the Queen of Heaven. Likewise, the sun in Egyptian mythology was called Sire and Osiris. In Sanskrit, it was called Aum; in Chaldean and Ethiopic it was called On; in Latinate languages it came to be known as Sol. These various names for the sun were combined into one name representing the highest wisdom in the personification, for example, of (Hebrew) King Solomon: Sol-Aum-On.[16]

Anderson also makes reference to the serpent as the spiraling motion of the celestial bodies as they move through the zodiac signs through the precession of the equinoxes.[17] At Aries, each of the twelve signs encompasses thirty, making the full 360 of the zodiac circle. Aries, which begins at the first point of right ascension of the Sun, goes from zero to thirty. According to Anderson, the term "right ascension" bears significance because RA (Right Ascension) is the name the Egyptians used to identify their "Sun God." Although exact dates for his reign are not completely known, they are believed to have fallen into the Age of Aries (4320–2160 BCE). It is likely that Ramses (or Ram-Isis) got his name as the holy keeper of the sacred light in this connection.[18]

According to Anderson, RAM (also lamb), the symbol used for Aries, is understood to be an acronym for right ascension meridian, where the sun appears annually around March 22, passes over the equinox, and emerges from winter into spring, symbolically from "death" into "life." While this association for RA and RAM works for modern

English, it may not apply to other languages. However, what Anderson says in the following excerpt implies a time when "the man from the east" spoke a language all men could understand. "It is the gate of gold, or Or, is a due east sign, and the knowledge . . . where the light which dispels the darkness came from the Or-i-ent, represented by Ab-ram, viz., Ab, original (or—first man) R.A.M.—or the original first right ascension of meridian, or man from the east, who spoke a language which all knew in the lands through which he travelled til he got into Egypt; viz., the sun language—the language of signs . . . "[19]

This gate of beginnings is not something that occurred only once in Earth's history; it only appears that way from the modern human perspective. Schwaller de Lubicz explains that the ancients' use of language was not so much to conceal as much as it was to reveal to those initiates trained with spiritual and astronomical understanding. They worked within a system that acknowledged "Creation" as one (not "the") starting point within an ongoing cycle of evolution within the time-space continuum.

Quoting Ampère, in *Essai sur la Philosophie des Sciences* (*Essai sur la Philosophie des Sciences*), Schwaller de Lubicz expresses the notion that science, equipped with the proper symbolic definitions, can better decipher original meanings. "[T]hese dogmas . . . often conceal ideas once reserved for a small number of initiates: and the secret of these ideas, though buried with them, can be rediscovered by those who study in depth all the types of ceremonies they prescribed. Hence, a science, given the names of 'the Symbolic' (the name I shall retain for it), proposes to uncover what was hidden behind such diverse emblems."[20]

Likewise, Anderson (1892) states that the "beast" in the Biblical Apocrypha (Book of Revelations) is nothing more than the ancients' description of the movement of the sun through the heavens: "Leo . . . is the beast alluded to in the Apocrypha, or Revelation of St. John . . . in whose house the Virgin Mer-I, or Mary, or Meré . . . had her home . . . The number of the beast . . . alludes to the sun rising at 6 am; 6 hours after it is mid-noon, and at 6 pm it sets, —3 sixes, 666."[21]

In a similar way, the word *altar* is a derivative of Al, El, Allah, and Elohim, from the Arabian, Hebraic, and Egyptian, respectively, names for "the central sun" and also the constellation Taurus (Tau)—*altau.* In the days before Moses, before the Ram (lamb) became the sacred animal, Taurus the bull was on the right ascension, that which was, astronomically speaking, "sitting at the right hand of God."[22]

Schwaller de Lubicz emphasizes that we find in Egypt a comprehensive system of knowledge rather than one still evolving. Their language was complete from the time of the earliest dynasties. As a result, we don't find conclusive evidence of ongoing research. Instead we see the application of a knowledge already possessed.[23]

Egyptologist and Pythagorean scholar John West, author of *Serpent in the Sky,* supports this sentiment. "Egyptian science, medicine, mathematics and astronomy were all of an exponentially higher order of refinement and sophistication than modern scholars will acknowledge. The whole of Egyptian civilization was based upon a complete and precise understanding of universal laws. And this profound understanding manifested itself in a consistent, coherent and inter-related system that fused science, art and religion into a single organic Unity . . . exactly the opposite of what we find in the world today."[24]

The universal laws to which John West is referring provide the landscape for a new understanding that can help us reconcile our past with the present and science with spirit. The evidence left by our ancient ancestors suggests they not only knew about the universal laws of nature, they became masters of those laws, particularly that of light technology, in both objective and subjective forms.

LIGHT TECHNOLOGY

Although the Great Pyramid in Egypt is most often the example that comes to mind, pyramids actually exist all over the world. The etymology of *pyramid,* which refers to the fourteenth and fifteenth century, gives the Latin *pirimidis* as well as the French *pyramide* (obelisk, stele). However, taking into consideration the Platonic connection of the tetrahedral shape with sacred fire and light, it seems likely that our modern word *pyre* may itself have come from the ancient structures.

Etymology for *pyre* mentions seventeenth-century Latin and Greek roots *pyra,* both having to do with sacrificial fires and altars.[25] As with every detail of ancient systems and structures, elements were used to symbolize deeper esoteric meaning. In this case, fire symbolized more than just the physical element; it referred to spiritual light or higher consciousness. We can also see a link to words having to do with anatomy, such as *pyrimidine* (a nucleic acid, as in DNA, a chemical compound important to several essential biochemical processes in the body). We can never know for sure whether there is a connection between our modern words and ancient worlds and practices.

Manly Hall alludes to the physical manifestation of light technology in the form of lamps the ancient priests were able to create, which would burn for centuries without replenishment. He explained how the ancient Romans used Hermetic methods to resolve gold into an oily substance that could burn.[26] These substances were used to keep tomb vaults lighted over long periods. Regarding Egyptian technology, British Rosicrucian and occult author Hargrave Jennings (1817–1890) collected many examples of times and places where the lamps had been found. In many of the cases, the lights were snuffed out as soon as the vaults were opened or they were broken into in some way that prevented the secret technology enabling their sustained light from being discovered. It is said one such lamp was discovered in the tomb of Cicero's daughter. It was still burning after more than fifteen centuries. It was also reported that when English monasteries were dissolved when Henry VIII left the Catholic Church that a small lamp was found, purportedly to have burned for nearly twelve centuries. Hall says two examples of these underground lamps are held in Leyden, Holland, at the Museum of Rarities, however, does not specify whether or not they are still burning.[27]

While this premise may seem impossibly "magical," we have a more recent example in the genius of Nikola Tesla (1856–1943), whose capabilities and discoveries seemed to tap into a type of "free energy." Well ahead of his time, Tesla's revolutionary work advanced electrical energy and contributed to the conveniences we take for granted today, such as wireless and remote technology, and fluorescent and neon lighting, to name a few. However, there are accounts of him conducting experiments with oscillators and generators that, had his work not been destroyed, might have produced an airship that could move in any direction without gas, wings, or propellers.[28] There are many instances throughout history of inventions that seemed outlandish for their time yet eventually science caught up and they were validated.

The ever-burning lamps of the ancients became the symbol for the eternal fire of the universe, reminding us to reflect on the more dogmatized use of terms by which we have been indoctrinated with religious and/or literal translations. In ancient Britain, Druid priests were purported to have started their altar fires by concentrating the sun's rays upon a specially cut crystal or aquamarine set in the form of a magic brooch that drew divine fire down from heaven. In certain temples, specially arranged lenses were located on the ceilings at various angles so that at the spring equinox each year the sun would send its rays through these lenses at high noon to light the altar fires.[29]

One of the reasons mistletoe was so revered as a sacred plant had to do with its ability to absorb cosmic light. Analogous to ancient Egyptian anatomists, Druids were also priests and physicians. They purportedly used magnetism to charge objects and amulets with universal healing powers as remedies. In light of the Druids' reverence for mistletoe and its magnetic quality, it has retained its reputation as a magical and magnetic plant to this day,[30] especially in Theosophical Medicine.

The ancient priests and Druids held sacred virtually every kind of life on Earth: plants, minerals, animals, and the human anatomy, aligned with the magnetic qualities each possessed. Moreover, they recognized this same magnetic quality within all of the planets, including Earth, which the ancient builders incorporated into their monuments.

While history tends to relegate these ancient practices to the fanciful, it is now time to explore the possibility that there was validity to their methods. Recall from chapter 3 that the word Greek word *mythos* originally referred to "historical accountings of ancient peoples," and was redefined in the Middle Ages by the Roman Church to mean "imaginative and fanciful tales."[31] It's important to keep in mind that within our modern languages there remains only a shadow of the original meaning, mostly because ancient languages were symbolic, and we've been indoctrinated into literal translations.

EGYPT'S LEGACY

Evidence pointing to the prior existence of advanced civilizations out of which the Egyptian system grew supports the greater antiquity of Egypt's legacy. West contends that while the actual physical location of an "Atlantis" may not presently be known, evidence exists of at least one highly advanced civilization predating the time of the Egyptian dynastic system by millennia.[32] When discussing the placement of the Pyramid's location, author Karl Anderson also supports the plausibility of an ancient "Atlantean" civilization that seeded Egyptian knowledge.

No maritime nation could navigate by chance; and that the Atlanteans were well versed in the mysteries of trigonometry and of solar, stellar, and lunar observations it is preposterous to deny. That the Phoenicians, who were colonists of the Atlanteans and who circumnavigated Africa, were also well informed in these particulars, is evident; and this is easily proved, inasmuch as the Great Pyramid is situated exactly on the ecliptic, and precisely covers by its angles the north, south, east, and west points, and the sun is exactly over it on the longest day of the year, viz., June 22. This, then, was a prime meridian or true right ascension every day at noon by the angle of the sun of the given day—or 90 high, on an equally divided day of twelve hours . . . [33]

During his twelve-year stay in Egypt, Schwaller de Lubicz studied the Great Pyramid, making observations that brought the question of Atlantis into the realm of geology, where evidence could be more easily assessed. He noted that the erosive pattern of the Sphinx Pyramid showed water erosion, not erosion by wind and sand. Moreover, other temples near the Sphinx showed the same water erosion. This distinction overturned the previously accepted chronology of the construction of the Sphinx, putting "orthodox" Egyptologists on the defensive. The predominance of water erosion meant that these monuments or temples were built prior to a biblical flood, which most scholars now believe occurred between 15,000 and 10,000 BCE.

Also supporting this date is researcher and author Graham Hancock; his computer simulations revealed that in 10,500 BCE Leo was the constellation rising in the east during the spring equinox at that time. That calculation means that the lion-bodied Sphinx, with its face oriented to the east, would have gazed directly into the Leo sun at the time of the spring equinox in that era.[34]

THE TEMPLE IS THE BODY

Although ancient monuments were built to reflect the movement of solar light and their orientation to it, they were also designed to mirror the human body temple. Manly Hall explained that it was a common practice among ancient civilizations to model their temples in the form of the human body. He cited such examples to include the Tabernacle of the Jews, the Egyptian Temple of Karnak, and religious structures in Hawaii. He also stated that many Christian structures were built to replicate the shape of a cross, so that the high altar is located in the church at the same place the brain occupies in the human body.[35]

In ancient Ayurveda, the crown chakra is located on the vertex of the skull, and is the place where spirit enters and exits the body "temple," as also described in scripture as Golgatha (place of the skull) from which spirit ascends and through which it descends. Hall surmises that this association may likely be the origin of our modern tradition about Saint Nicholas, "Sinter Clas," or Santa Claus, that has him entering through the chimney, especially given the fact that his place of origin is the North Pole aligned with the North Star. The North Star has always been associated with immortality because it is "circumpolar" and therefore always visible from Earth; it never sets (dies) along the ecliptic.[36]

Leonardo da Vinci's *Vitruvian Man* shows that the crucifix, or cross, not only refers to the four elements and directions, it also symbolizes the human body: head north, feet south, and arms east and west. It also represents the Fibonacci number, or phi, in its anatomical ratios therein represented.

Supposing that Hall and Anderson are correct in their assertion that ancient texts have more to do with astronomical and anatomical correlations, we might view the aspect of initiation involving travel to the underworld differently. In ancient Egypt, the adepts were led through the underworld called Amenti, a place associated with the setting of the sun and the westerly direction. Also called the "Land of the West," it was known as the place where the God Ra traveled during the night. The Goddess Amentet was a guide for those souls entering the underworld, but she was also known as a goddess of fertility and rebirth who nourished the travelers with food and water.[37]

The ancient mystery schools taught that the human body has three major regions, analogous to the three worlds of heaven, earth, and hell. In anatomical correlation, the physical location for "hell" rests at the base of the spine, where the sleeping serpent must awaken and enter the higher portals associated with heavenly mansions along the spine (as in kundalini). Between heaven and hell is earth (that which Scandinavians call Midgard or Middle Garden and the Chinese call jiang guo). The land at the middle, or the Middle Kingdom, is halfway between heaven and earth) and assigned to that region of the body where digestion and the churning of superior and inferior energies take place. Chinese medicine employs the terms *Upper, Middle, and Lower (Triple) Burners* to refer to the body's three regions, assigning one of the twelve meridians the name "Triple Burner," or San Jiao. Below is the region of darkness, where, by way of either the reproductive act or excretion, we experience the necessity of letting go.

By correspondence, in Egyptian mysticism there are three principles known as "uas," "ankh," and "djed." *Uas* stood for the act of creation, which simultaneously gave birth to the existence of evil, or rather the act of separation. *Ankh* represents the giver of life, whence both principles of spirit and body exist. The knot of the ankh is what will bring life to "uas" when connected to the third principle, djed, represented by the column.[38]

The column (*djed*) becomes the symbol of support and stability to the corporeal state, uniting spirit, soul and body, analogous to the spinal column along which kundalini flows. It unites the four elements through the weaving of the knot of the ankh, shown horizontally, tying east and west polarities together. Thus, the ankh became an extremely sacred instrument used by priests in Egyptian ceremony.[39]

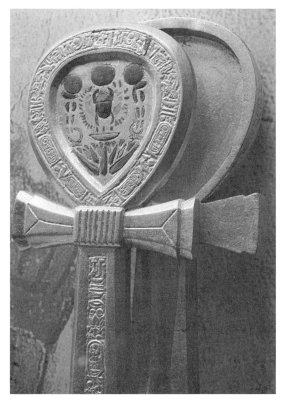

Fig. 6.4. The Egyptian ankh.

Schwaller de Lubicz writes that the covered temple (or dome) represented the skull, and the northern (positive) end of the spinal column.[40] In the Gospels of the Christian scriptures, this place was described as the upper room where Jesus sat with his disciples. The brain and its twelve cortical convolutions, as well as the sun and the twelve constellations revolving around it, are symbolic of this upper room.

In the same manner that the twelve disciples gathered around Jesus in the holy of holies and were later sent out to preach the Gospel, the convolutions gather around the central opening (third ventricle) in the brain, using the nervous system to send messages to the body below. By definition, it sounds like the description of the serpent symbol, which was a recurring theme with ancient anatomists. They described it as "a twisting together; a turn, a twist, or coil," and "a rolled up or coiled condition," "a turn of anything coiled; whorl."

These convolutions match our earlier description of the curling and coiling surface of the brain's cortex and its ability, together with the presence of neuromelanin, to conduct light and electromagnetic energy that enhances one's inner sight and the ability to see other dimensions.

The third ventricle of the brain, also known as the "vaulted chamber" of initiation, is the place from which the consecrated saints' auras are represented to emanate the halo. Around it sit three anthropomorphic "kings": the pituitary gland, the pineal gland, and the optic thalamus.[41] The Hindus refer to the third ventricle of the brain as the Cave of Brahma. Many esoteric traditions refer to it as the seat of the soul, where life-force energy culminates after traveling from the base of the spine up to the brain.[42] The flow of energy that arises from this practice is experienced as a serpentine undulation motion. This motion is similar to that of a serpent moving energy from the base of the spine up to the brain, affecting an awakening of consciousness described as "spiritual baptism." This can be seen as the equivalent of "being born again," a sacred tradition described since antiquity.[43]

INITIATION AND
THE ASTROLOGICAL BODY

In *Brahmandic Gyanum,* author Vashist Vaid explains that the seven planetary chains in our solar system act like energy distribution centers containing a total of forty-nine rounds and sub-rounds.[44] Eastern mysticism teaches that there are correspondingly forty-nine (seven times seven) sacred nerve centers within the body, as well as the seven major energy centers along the spine known as the chakras or wheels of energy.[45]

Anderson explains that planets are endowed with immense magnetic power, interacting with one another, larger ones upon smaller ones, and imparting certain magnetic qualities onto the human form: "Man being a universe in himself, and capable of great magnetic powers by which to attract and repel others, he also is ruled by these signs in twelve divisions of his body, corresponding to the twelve divisions of the zodiac . . . "[46]

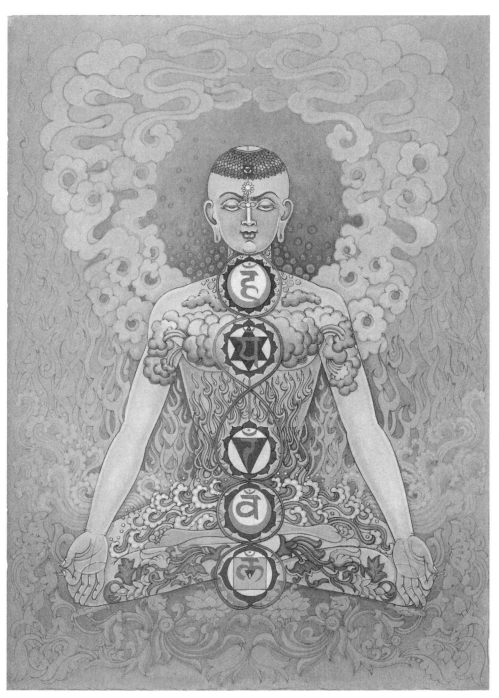

Fig. 6.5. Seven energy centers along the spine.
Painting by Pieter Weltevrede from *Chakras* by Harish Johari.

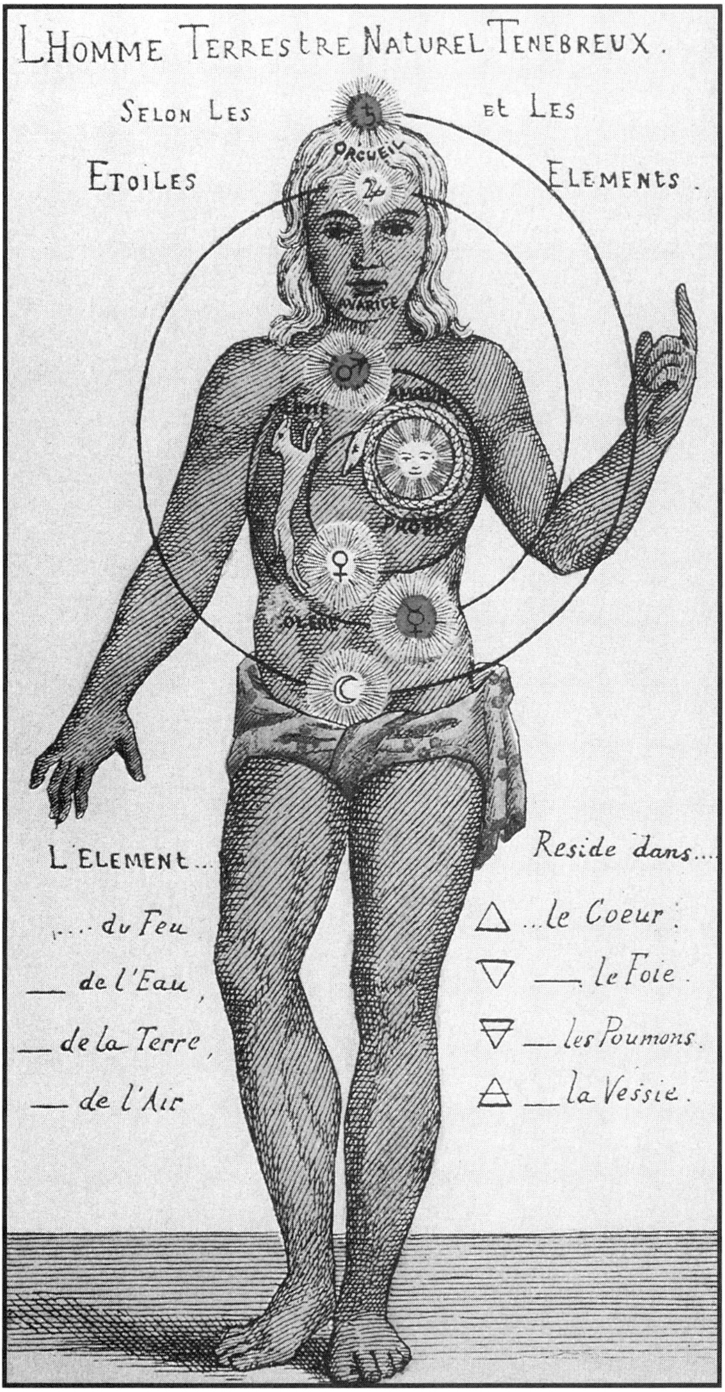

Fig. 6.6. Planets, organs, and elements in ancient anatomy. From Dover Pictura.

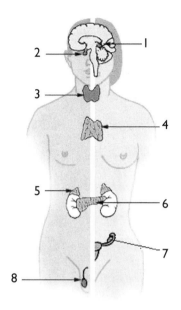

Fig. 6.7. Location of the endocrine glands. (Note the similarity between the planets in fig. 6.6 and the organs in fig. 6.7. In 6.7, the kidneys are each assigned a number; however, in 6.6 the same planet rules over both kidneys as one unit.)

Each sign of the zodiac corresponds to a part of the body and shares governance with the chakras and endocrine glands as well (as depicted in figs. 6.6, 6.7, and 6.8). In *Western Astrology and Chinese Medicine*, author Jonathan Clogstoun-Willmott associates the twelve meridians with the twelve signs:[47]

Lung – Aries

Large intestine – Taurus

Stomach – Gemini

Spleen – Cancer

Heart – Leo

Small intestine – Virgo

Urinary bladder – Libra

Kidney – Scorpio

Pericardium – Sagittarius

San Jiao (Triple Burner) – Capricorn

Gallbladder – Aquarius

Liver – Pisces

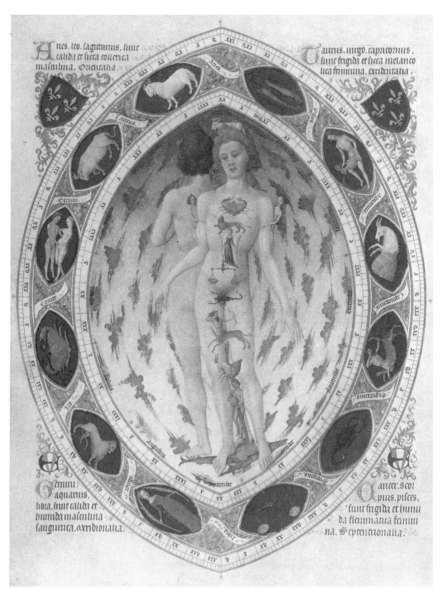

Fig. 6.8. Depiction of astrological anatomy. From Dover Pictura.

Two of the organs most active in the link among planets and the energetic body are, according to Hall, the spleen and the liver—gateways through which the invisible world interacts with physical anatomy.[48] In Oriental medicine, each organ acts as a gateway between the visible and invisible realm and is responsible for relaying energy in a synergistic relationship with other organs that together maintain overall health. These include correlations between and among specific planets, seasons, sounds, color, and emotions.

Of particular interest to certain planetary correspondences are the spinal column, endocrine system, and chakras, shown in figure 6.5, a Hindu depiction of the "planetary human body."

THE SERPENTINE SPINE

Just as the Earth has its axis mundi, the spinal column behaves as an axis for the human body, conducting electromagnetic energies between

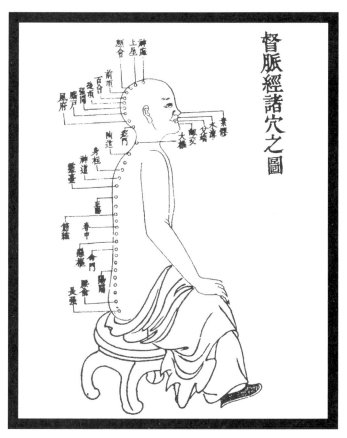

Fig. 6.9. Chinese depiction of the energy that runs along the spinal column. From Dover Pictura.

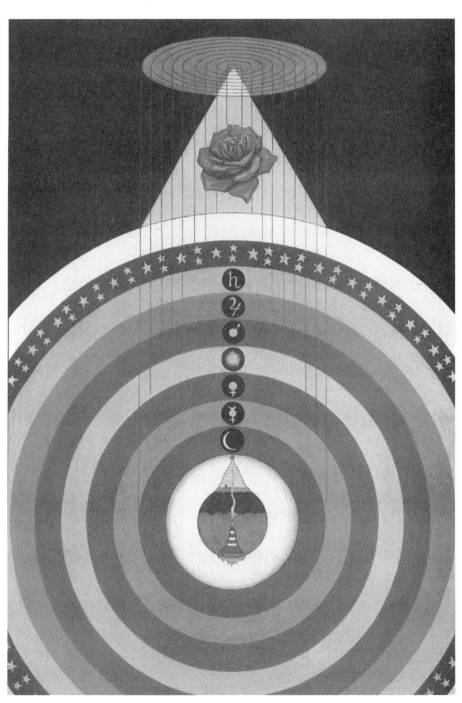

Fig. 6.10. Earth's "spinal column" (axis mundi) along which Earth
and celestial energies flow. From Dover Pictura.

heaven and earth. The cerebral spinal fluid is analogous to a river that carries nourishment to the neural structures and tissues.

The spine has always played a significant role in the religious symbolism of the ancients, often being referred to as a wand, scepter, or serpent, and sometimes as a ladder, winding road, or stairway. In the Hindu religion three canals in the spinal system are known as the *ida, pingala,* and *sushumna;* they connect lower generative centers with the brain. The Greeks used the caduceus and winged staff of Hermes, which consisted of a long rod (central sushumna) and ended in a knob

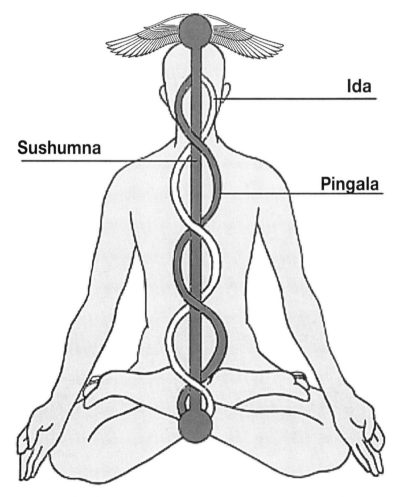

Fig. 6.11. Hindu *ida, pingala,* and *sushumna* along the spine, with serpent spiral and wings representing left and right hemispheres of the brain.

or ball (analogous to the pons of the medulla oblongata of the brain). On each side of the knob are wings that represent the two lobes of the cerebrum. In this representation, along the staff and twisted around it, are two serpents, one black, the other white, representing the feminine and masculine energies.[49]

The frontal cortex of the skull (corresponding to frontal sinus) is located behind the eyes and just above the nose. In this location jewels are placed on the foreheads of Buddhas.

It is also the point from which the serpent arose from the crowns of ancient Egyptians. Figure 6.13 provides an example of the Hindu Shiva's third eye. Mystical schools teach that this location is the seat of Jehovah in the human body,[50] where the male and female "serpent energies" (kundalini) rise up along the spine and flower into higher consciousness, or decision-making, at the third eye (pineal) or "eye single" from the Christian scriptures. Indeed, Matthew 6:22 (King James Version) tells us: "The light of the body is the eye; if therefore thine eye be single, thy whole body shall be filled with light."

The initiation process of ancient Eygpt was intended to reestablish the function of the pineal gland and its connection to the pituitary gland so that the individual could then perceive the invisible realms.

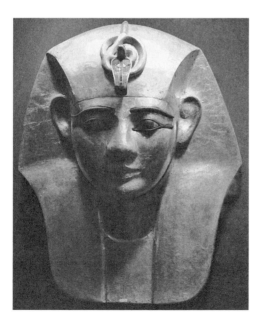

Fig. 6.12. Mask of Amenemope, a pharoah from Egypt's Twenty-First Dynasty. Photograph by John Campana (CC BY-SA 2.0).

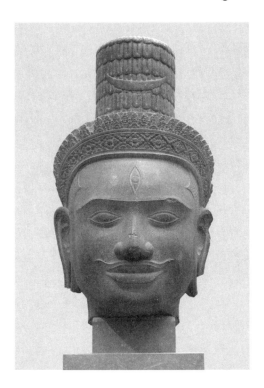

Fig. 6.13. A Cambodian sculpture of Shiva with the third eye.

The importance of this relationship between the pituitary and pineal glands cannot be overstated. The entire hormonal-glandular system holds tremendous power over biological processes, and the connection between the pineal gland and pituitary gland clearly supports clinical psychologist Dr. Edward Bynum's research on the role of neuromelanin to access subtle energy and light.

THE ENDOCRINE SYSTEM

The pineal gland, which sits in the geometric center of the cerebral cortex (the vaulted chamber as stated above), was understood to be the location of the single eye or the Eye of Horus. (Please see fig. 6.15). In its shape it resembles that of a pinecone, which is featured in art and architecture around the globe. The largest of these examples can be found in the Vatican Square in Rome (see fig. 6.17). Moreover, this gland secretes an oil much like the resin secreted by pinecones. Author

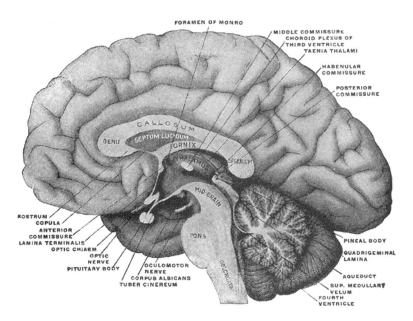

Fig. 6.14. Sagittal view of the brain and pineal gland (or pineal body). Note the resemblance to the Eye of Horus shown below in figure 6.15. From Dover Pictura.

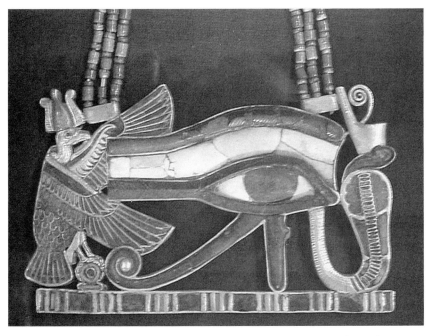

Fig. 6.15. Eye of Horus pendant. Photograph by Jon Bodsworth.

David Wilcock writes: "the word 'pineal' comes from the Latin *pinea,* which means pine cone. Ancient cultures all over the world were fascinated by the pine cone and pineal-gland-shaped images, and consistently used them in their highest forms of spiritual artwork. Pythagoras, Plato, Iamblichus, Descartes and others wrote of this gland with great reverence. It has been called the seat of the soul."[51]

Fig. 6.16. Close-up of the pineal gland. From Dover Pictura.

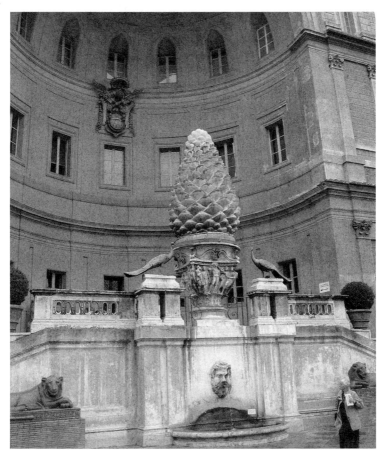

Fig. 6.17. Bronze pigna (pinecone) at the Vatican.
Photograph by Lance Mountain (CC BY-SA 2.0).

The pine in terms of botanical history predates deciduous plants, dating back to the Precambrian period on Earth two hundred million years ago.

In *Esoteric Healing*, volume IV, Alice Bailey (1880–1949) addresses the importance of the portals within the endocrine system: "There is . . . the awakening of these centres through the process of initiation. This . . . only happens when the man is consciously upon the Path . . . The centres determine the man's point of evolution . . . they work directly upon the physical body through the medium of the endocrine system."[52]

The endocrine system includes the pituitary, pineal, thyroid, thymus, adrenals, germinal cells of Leydig, and the gonads: seven organs in all. Although some systems disagree on planetary assignment, all agree that these seven ductless endocrine glands have a relationship with the seven original planets. One system assigns this correlation: pituitary–Jupiter, pineal–Moon, thyroid–Venus, thymus–Saturn, adrenals–Mercury, Leydig–Sun, and gonads–Mars.[53]

THE CHAKRA SYSTEM

Just as the seven planets are viewed as energy distribution centers, so too are the chakras viewed as wheels of energy located within the body, as discussed earlier. As is the case with most disciplines, variations exist in the assignment of planetary bodies to the specific energetic chakras. A basic overview of the chakras is offered here.[54]

- The root chakra, Muladhara, is located at the base of the spine, and is associated with the earth element and qualities of being stable or being challenged with survival issues.
- The second chakra, Svadhisthana, is located at the sacral plexus, and is associated with the water element and emotional attachments.
- The third chakra, Manipura, is located at the solar plexus, and is associated with the fire element and issues related to self-esteem and empowerment.
- The fourth chakra, Anahata, is located at the heart, and is

associated with the air element and the ability to show compassion and love.

- The fifth chakra, Vishuddha, is located at the throat, and is associated with the ether element and the ability to communicate one's knowledge, wisdom, and truth.
- The sixth chakra, Ajna, is located between the eyes (the third eye). It has no element association, and relates to spiritual vision.
- The seventh chakra, Sahasrara, is located at the crown of the head. It has no element association, and relates to unity, integration of body and spirit, enlightenment.

Whether Egyptian, Indian, or Chinese, ancient cultural systems agree that there are correspondences among human anatomy and our solar planetary system. As a civilization we are now experiencing the effects of centuries where the practice of separation has nearly paralyzed a deeper desire for unity. Through the misuse and misinterpretation of language, we have forgotten the body's sacred connections to the universe and to cosmic light.

Perhaps by revisiting these sacred sciences we can recall that darkness and light are inextricably connected. Rather than running away from that which arises from the dark unknown, we can remember that the greater the darkness, the greater our capacity to receive and conduct light. This concept may be seen as analogous to deep-sea dwelling creatures like the giant squid, whose eyes are as large as a human head in order to absorb sufficient light for them to navigate through the darkness.

The new technology needed is that which unites the two eyes into the "eye single" so that we are able to cultivate light that can penetrate the darkness. Instead of viewing conflict and strife as fearful, they may be viewed instead as opportunities to facilitate more light. They can be perceived as messengers, just as symptoms show up in the body to remind us when we are out of balance. If we maintain a polarized perception, we are, as the observers, creating more of that polarization in our world. On the other hand, if we can embrace the darkness with an attitude of allowing the "return of the prodigal son," we become facilitators of healing instead.

7

PHI-LOSOPHY
The Mean between the Extremes

This chapter continues with exploration of the correspondences we find between the microcosm and macrocosm. We see that an underlying key connection, which unifies these parts within the context of the whole (cosmos), reveals itself through a particular number. The language of numbers (mathematics) provides one motif for virtually all subjects in our culture, such as art, music, architecture, and science. For the purpose of this discussion it is necessary to examine numbers as the ancient mathematicians applied them. This discussion begins with a look at rational and irrational numbers, and a determination of how their meanings might correspond in philosophy. We will then discover how phi (ϕ) (an irrational number) came to be known through Pythagorean concepts, revealing itself in geometry, music, and astronomy.

FINDING VALUE IN THE IRRATIONAL

To duplicate or not to duplicate, that is the question (or at least one fundamental question). Rational numbers are those that can be written as a fraction, such as 5 becoming 5/1, or 0.75 becoming ¾, or 1.75 becoming 7/4. Rational numbers provide patterns that are repeatable. It is interesting that *rational* is also a term we use to describe a particular thought process as being logical and reasonable. Irrational numbers, on the other hand, cannot be expressed as a fraction or quotient between two integers. They can only be expressed by decimals, whereby the numbers that follow the decimal point never cease and never duplicate; they continue on into infinity. Examples of irrational numbers are the well-known Pi (π)—3.1415926 . . . and Phi (ϕ)—1.618033 . . . or phi (lower case) 0.618033 . . . There was in recent memory some popular recognition of Pi on March 14, 2015, the number of which date expresses the first five digits (and the ancient date that Julius Caesar was prophesied to "beware").

As unique and complex as these numbers may be—they are not uncommon in nature and the cosmos. There is always at least one irrational number found in between two rational numbers. When irrational and rational numbers are combined they produce another irrational number.[1] From a philosophical standpoint, it would seem that rationality (expressing an identical concept or relationship) does not necessarily support creativity. On the other hand, an irrational number serves to create a new variable, so perhaps an irrational concept could also lead to a new solution—begging the question: Is it always reasonable to be rational?

Scientist David Bohm (1917–1992) believed there to be a creative process inherent in science that science itself may have forgotten. He and coauthor F. David Peat (a holistic physicist) advocated for renewed emphasis on ideas rather than formulas, and on meaning rather than mechanics, in their 1987 book *Science, Order, and Creativity.* They also emphasized the importance of looking at the whole rather than only one fragmentary part to perform analysis. While true that one can glean from any part (microcosm) some information regarding the whole (macrocosm), it remains questionable as to whether any fragment may be defined as the whole in its entirety. There is always a greater or smaller part, cycle, or dimension to explore.

Likewise, there is much more to any subject than what is merely repeatable and obvious. Since irrational numbers are always present amidst rational numbers it suggests that rationality may not provide the final or complete answer regarding the whole. To derive complete meaning from any given situation or subject, one must consider both perspectives. Both types of numbers have ratio in common. Defining ratio and proportion is the next step in the process of understanding the importance of the irrational number phi (φ), to which Plato referred as "the mean between the extremes."[2]

UNDERSTANDING RATIO AND PROPORTION

Ratio (logos), which in Greek means "word, thought or reason" is a way to measure the quantitative differences between two different items or integers (a and b).[3] The formula used to describe ratio is written a:b, whereby when a is divided by b, it describes a relationship between the two. A simple example would be to substitute the number 4 for a, and the number 2 for b, so that the formula is 4:2 and would be translated as: 4 (a) is twice the size of 2 (b).[4]

Proportion (analogia), from whence comes the word *analogy,* describes the measure of equivalence between two ratios. There are two types of proportions, *discontinuous* and *continuous.* Discontinuous relates two completely separate sets of variables to one another: A:B::C:D, or 2:4::7:14, such that the equivalent measure between the two sets is ½: 2 is to 4 as 7 is to 14. However, A and B do not in any way define what C and D could be, because there are any number of possibilities that would work. So discontinuous proportion is not especially unique.

Continuous proportion, described in the formula A:B::B:C is such that when A and B are known, we can determine what C will be. There is a direct link from A to B and from B to C, thus continuous. A numerical example of this link might be 2:4::4:8, for instance, so that each new variable may be absolutely determined as long as A and B are identified. Thus, continuous proportion is a much more facile formula to employ when the goal is to define specific relations, because the common link among all variables is a number (in this example 4) rather than the proportional relationship (½).[5] In this example of continuous proportion, 4 is the "mean between" 2 and 8.

So far, the examples given involve measurement between two ratios with three or four variables. In the first example, we have four variables (A, B, C, D) such that the first two cannot determine the second two.

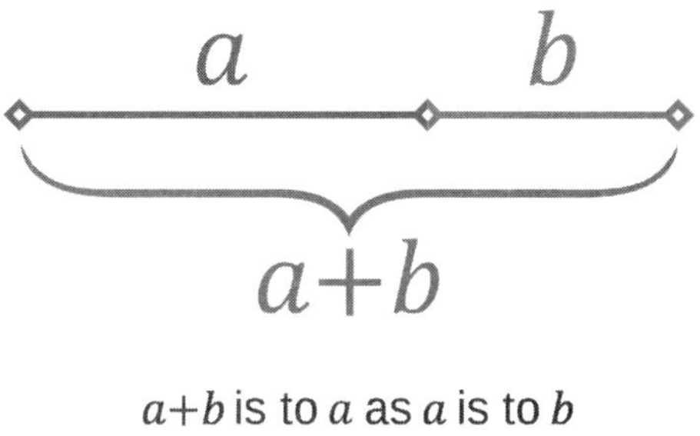

$$a \qquad b$$

$$a+b$$

a+b is to a as a is to b

Fig. 7.1. Golden ratio or golden proportion.

In the second example we have three variables (A, B, C) such that the third variable will determine all subsequent variables. Ancient mathematicians pondered whether any true proportion exists that only involves two variables.

Recalling that the definition of proportion must involve two sets of ratios, it serves no purpose to write a formula like A:B::B:A (A is to B exactly as it is to itself). Such a relation represents only one ratio (the relationship between A and B). However, the formula that does work using only two variables is A:B::B:A + B; A is to B as B is to the sum of A and B. This sentence describes two different relationships with only two variables.

The smaller segment, B, relates to the longer segment A in the same way that the longer segment A relates to the sum of both shorter and longer segments: A + B. It can also be written thus: A + B:A::A:B. This approach is how the ancients discovered the golden proportion (aka golden mean, or golden section), which is the irrational number Phi/phi ɸ (1.618 . . . /0.618 . . .).[6]

EXPRESSION OF UNITY

A remarkable quality about this golden proportion is that it expresses unity while creating infinitely in both smaller and larger proportions. In the example shown in figure 7.1, unity has been divided into two segments, both of which mathematically relate back to the whole in a truly proportional sense. Further division by Phi/phi, however, produces an infinite number of variables that all relate back to unity . . . quite a paradox! "That proportion . . . happens to equal the irrational number known as . . . 0.618 . . . or 1:1.618 . . . Phi . . . an apt expression for the transcendence of humankind, and also gives us the ability to understand how it is possible that the unified universe can be divided into myriad forms, yet continuously relate back to the ever-present unity of all things."[7]

This marvel corresponds to Pythagorean philosophy (circa the sixth century BCE) where the study of numbers took on a mystical component, linking it with geometry, music, and astronomy, and taught within the context of philosophy. According to author Mario Livio, it was Hippasus of Metapontum who was given credit for having discovered phi, but he actually learned it from Pythagoras while a member of the Pythagorean Brotherhood.[8] As an initiate, he had been sworn to secrecy and ultimately violated that trust. Iamblichus (245–325), founder of the Syrian School of Neoplatonism, gives this account: "It is related of Hippasus that he was a Pythagorean, and that, owing to his being the first to publish and describe the sphere from the twelve pentagons, he perished at sea for his impiety, but he received credit for the discovery, though really it all belonged to HIM (for in this way they refer to Pythagoras, and they do not call him by his name)."[9]

Livio explains that the "sphere from the twelve pentagons" refers to the dodecahedron, one of the platonic solids discussed in previous chapters, which is intimately connected to the golden ratio (see figs. 7.2 and 7.3). Plato was himself a Pythagorean and, in addition to Pythagoras, was one of the most influential minds ultimately impacting Western Civilization. We will return a little later to him in this chapter.

Pythagoras (571–495 BCE) has remained a quasi-mythical figure. Written accounts about his life came from his followers, including Plato. Pythagoras himself felt that knowledge was an ever-evolving process that written words served only to limit.[10] His biographers all agree that he traveled extensively at an early age to assimilate the knowledge of the ancients, studying the longest in Egypt (twenty-two years), with time also spent in Babylon and the Orient. After a brief return to his

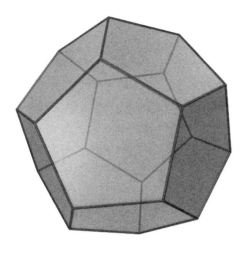

Fig. 7.2. Dodecahedron with pentagon face. Created by Cyp (CC BY-SA 3.0).

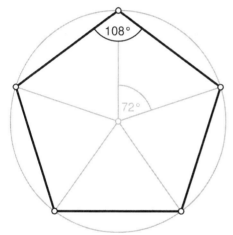

Fig. 7.3. Pentagon showing the golden ratio; two quantities (72 and 108) are in the golden ratio if their ratio is the same as the ratio of their sum to the larger of the two quantities. 72 is to 108 (72+36) as 108 is to 180 (108+72). Illustration by László Németh.

home on the island of Samos, he became discouraged by the political tyranny of Polycrates and settled in Croton, Italy, when he was in his forties (around 530 BCE). There he established a school of science and philosophy.[11]

PYTHAGOREAN PHILOSOPHY OF NUMBER

Quite different from today's predominantly quantitative mathematics, Pythagoras's approach to numbers was a living, qualitative reality that required experiential learning. Whereas contemporary math uses numbers as symbols to denote known quantities, Pythagoras believed that number should be discovered rather than used.[12] Pythagoreans emphasized the notion of divine number and harmonia, "intent on unifying all levels of human experience through the principles of harmony."[13] Credited for having coined both the words *philosophy* ("lover of wisdom"), and *mathematics* ("that which is learned"), Pythagoras and his followers emphasized the concept of order in all things. Mathematics was applied for the purpose of discovering order in ethics, geometry, music, and the cosmos (for which the Greek word *kosmos* actually means order). This application is evident in the four branches of Pythagorean study of number.[14]

Arithmetic – number in itself
Geometry – number in space
Music of harmonics – number in time
Astronomy – number in space and time

PYTHAGOREAN THEORY

I swear by the discoverer of the Tetraktys
Which is the spring of all our wisdom
The perennial fount and root of Nature.

PYTHAGOREAN OATH[15]

One of the most important images to Pythagoreans was the tetraktys. It symbolically represents each of the branches mentioned above. Regarding arithmetic (number in itself), the tetraktys reveals the perfection of number and represents unity with the number 1 at the apex (see figs. 7.4A, B, and C). Author Guthrie explains: "the Tetraktys itself represents the vertical hierarchy of relation between Unity and emerging Multiplicity."[16] The number 1 becomes 2; 2 becomes 3; 3 becomes 4; 4 becomes many; and when these numbers are added up (1+2+3+4) the sum is 10, creating the image of the tetraktys, and another cycle of unity symbolized by the 10.

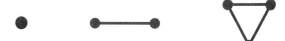

Fig. 7.4A. Progression from one dot to formation of the tetrahedron. 1 becomes 2; 2 becomes 3; 3 becomes 4. The sum of all equals 10 (perfect number).

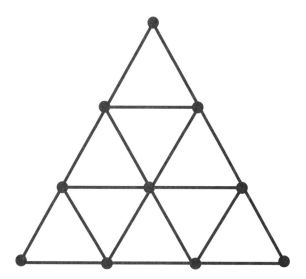

Fig. 7.4B. Tetraktys with ten dots.

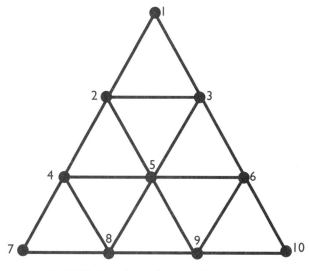

Fig. 7.4C. Tetraktys shown with numbers.

GEOMETRY: NUMBER IN SPACE

Regarding geometry, the Pythagorean triangle remains the fundamental image (fig. 7.5). According to Livio, a 1940 book titled *The Pythagorean Proposition* by Elisha Scott Loomis presented 367 proofs of the Pythagorean theorem, some of which included those by Leonardo da Vinci during the Italian Renaissance. On an ancient Babylonian clay tablet, referred to as "Plimpton 322," accounts of what is now known as Pythagorean triples were discovered. It reveals three common integers [3, 4, 5] that satisfy the Pythagorean theorem.[17]

The Pythagorean theorem states that the squared length of the hypotenuse (longest side of a right-angled triangle) equals the sum of the squares of the two shorter sides, $h^2 = a^2 + b^2$ (or $a^2 + b^2 = c^2$ as in fig. 7.6).

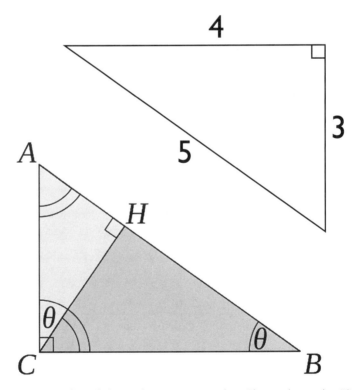

Fig. 7.5. Examples of the Pythagorean triangles. Above shows the "3-4-5 triangle" and below is the Pythagorean triangle showing its relationship to phi.

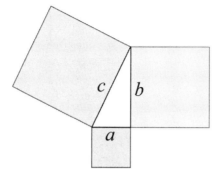

Fig. 7.6. The sum of areas a plus b (shown as squares) equals the area of the square of c (hypotenuse side of triangle). If we were to assign a + b the numbers 3 and 4, the formula would be: $3^2 + 4^2 = 5^2$ (9 + 16 = 25). By Wapcaplet (CC BY-SA 3.0).

MUSIC: NUMBER IN TIME

To understand the application of number on music and harmonics, Pythagoras experimented with the monochord (which he is also credited with having invented). The monochord is a one-stringed instrument with a moveable bridge. He discovered that dividing a string by consecutive numbers creates harmonious sounds called consonant intervals. When two random notes are played together, it results in a dissonant (non-harmonious) sound. In this way he discovered harmonic progression and the musical scale.[18]

In music, unison is achieved when the strings are of equal length, creating a ratio 1:1. Pythagoras discovered that when he moved the bridge to the midway point on the string, the musical octave is created by the ratio 1:2. A perfect fifth is created with the ratio 2:3 and the perfect fourth with the ratio 3:4.[19] (See fig. 7.9.) This relationship is also depicted in the image of the tetraktys with dots, which reveals these ratios line by line, starting at the top: (line)1:(line)2, the octave; 2:3, the perfect fifth; and 3:4, the perfect fourth.[20] Guthrie explains that the overtone series provides the "architectural foundation of the musical scale, the basic 'field' of which is the octave, 1:2, or the doubling of the vibrational frequency."[21] (See table 7.1.)

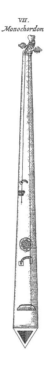

VII.
Monochordon

Fig. 7.7. The monochord instrument. By Athanasius Kircher, *Musurgia Universalis* (1650) book VI, chapter II, plate 8, between pages 486 and 487.

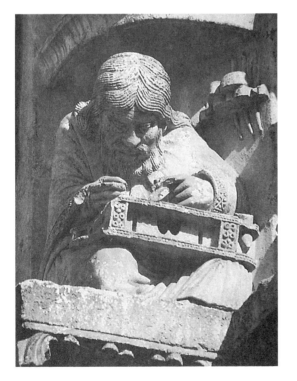

Fig. 7.8. From the Chartres Cathedral in Notre Dame; carving depicts a philosopher (believed to be Pythagoras) playing a monochord. Photograph by Jean-Louis Lascoux.

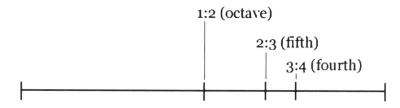

Fig. 7.9. Mathematical ratios of the musical intervals that are consonant (in harmony) with the whole string and each other.

TABLE 7.1. PYTHAGOREAN SCALE SHOWING RATIOS, INTERVALS, AND HARMONIC PROPORTIONS

Note	Ratio	Music Interval	Proportion
C (low)	1/1	Unison	6
D	9/8	Major second	
E			
F	4/3	Perfect fourth	8
G	3/2	Perfect fifth	9
A			
B			
C (high)	2/1	Octave	12

Source: Adapted from Guthrie, *The Pythagorean Sourcebook and Library*, p. 327.

The Pythagorean scale describes how the two extremes of the low C (1) and the high C (2) are connected and unified through the harmonic proportions that mediate between the two.

This unification of the opposites was central to Pythagorean philosophy and is described by the terms *pera,* referring to form or boundary, and *apeira,* referring to indefinite matter. To *pera* Pythagoreans ascribed odd numbers, and to *apeira* they ascribed even numbers. Once again, the tetraktys was the symbol Pythagoreans used to express this mathematical relationship. It was also later revealed by Plato in *Timaeus,* where it was referred to as the Lambda Tetraktys (see fig. 7.10). The Lambda Tetraktys also became known as the symbol for Plato's "World Soul" in that it describes numerically and musically, through the derivation of arithmetic and harmonic means, how the Demiurge mediates between, and unifies, the extremes. With even numbers on one side, and odd on the other, the even numbers give harmonic ratios when addition is applied, and the odd numbers when multiplication is applied. Using this formula within the context of the octave, we are able to derive the harmonic mean of the fifth when applying addition, and that of the fourth when applying multiplication.

To best explain how a harmonic mean occurs using the Lambda Tetraktys, Guthrie substitutes 6:12 for the two extremes of the octave (1:2) ratio of string division.[22] When we apply addition, 6 and 12 become 18. To get the mean, we divide by 2, which produces 9. The number 9 (note G) is in a 2:3 ratio to 6 (low C octave tone) and produces the perfect fifth interval. When we multiply those same numbers (6 × 12) and multiply by 2 we get 144. In this case we divide 144 by the sum of the octave extremes (6 + 12 = 18) to get 8. The ratio of 6:8 is also 3:4, represented by the perfect fourth (low C to F).

Providing a discourse on music theory is not the primary objective of this chapter. It serves our purpose simply to show how the mathematical formulas were used by Pythagoras to create the musical scale, and to show music's relationship to Phi (1.618...)/phi (0.618...).

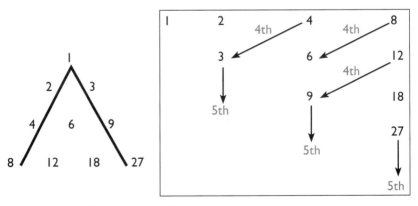

Fig. 7.10. Lambda Tetraktys. On the left are even numbers, representing the indefinite, and on the right are odd numbers, representing form or boundaries. The number 3^3 (cubed) is 27, representing form and three-dimensional reality represented by the geometric cube.

Instead of the monochord, we will use the piano keyboard to demonstrate the presence of the golden ratio. This approach allows us to also see the connection between phi and the Fibonacci number sequence: 0, 1, 1, 2, 3, 5, 8, 13, 21, 34, 55, and so on. In this sequence, the two previous numbers determine the next number in the sequence: $0 + 1 = 1$, $1 + 1 = 2$, $1 + 2 = 3$, $2 + 3 = 5$, $3 + 5 = 8$, $5 + 8 = 13$, $8 + 13 = 21$, $13 + 21 = 34$, and so forth.

After the eighth sequence ($13 + 21 = 34$), the constant ratio that appears when dividing the smaller number by the larger is phi, 0.618 ($34/55 = 0.618$), and when you divide the larger by the smaller, it yields 1.618. This ratio is easier to see on a piano, because within an octave, there are 8 white keys and 5 black keys, totaling 13 in all (see fig. 7.11). The fifth white note is called the "dominant" because it is the eighth key within the entire scale, and 8/13 produces a ratio in approximation to phi 0.61538. In Western musical composition the dominant note (particularly when immediately preceded by the tonic note in a sequence of this duo) signifies that the musical piece is ended. Both the fourth and fifth intervals were considered "perfect" because, unlike other intervals that may be minor or major, the fourth and fifth are considered stable, as are the unison and octave. As we move on to the subject of astronomy, we will see the significance of the musical scale and intervals with regard to Pythagorean philosophy of the cosmos.

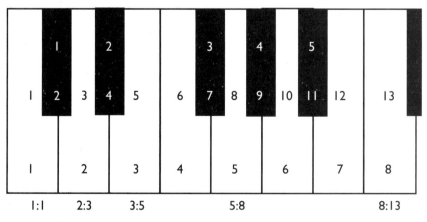

Fig. 7.11. The piano keyboard is based upon Fibonacci numbers, with five black keys and eight white keys, adding up to thirteen.

ASTRONOMY:
NUMBER IN SPACE AND TIME

In Pythagorean astronomy, once again we see that the tetraktys becomes useful in revealing the process of manifestation in the universe. One represents the point, two represents the line, three represents the surface, and four represents the first three-dimensional form through the tetrahedron. In *The Pythagorean Sourcebook and Library,* Kenneth Guthrie includes an account by Theon of Smyrna, taken from *Mathematics Useful for Understanding Plato,* chapter 38 (translated by Robert and Deborah Lawlor).

Theon of Smyrna explained that there is more than one tetraktys (also called quarternary). In fact, there are eleven in total, one of which was just discussed pertaining to musical ratios, the fourth of which pertains to the four elements (as in fig. 7.12), in order of most subtle to least subtle. Fire (1) heat; air (2) moist; water (3) cold; earth (4) dry.[23] This correspondence is consistent with the nature of the elements when they combine to produce changes in the atmosphere, and in the body through the four humors. When combining 1 and 2 (heat with moisture) we have air; when combining 2 and 3 (moisture with cold) we get water; when combining 3 and 4 (cold with dry), we get earth.

Regarding the fifth quarternary, Theon of Smyrna explains that the elements also have specific shapes (later known as the platonic solids): fire takes the shape of a pyramid (also referred to as the tetrahedron); air the octahedron; water the icosahedron; and earth the cube.[24] (Centuries later, these correspondences became the basis for Kepler's laws of planetary motion, mentioned in chapter 5). Regarding unity and number, Theon of Smyrna had this to say: "Unity is the principle of all things and the most dominant of all that is: all things emanate from it and it emanates from nothing. It is indivisible and it is everything in power. It is immutable and never departs from its own nature through multiplication ($1 \times 1 = 1$). Everything that is intelligible and not yet created exists in it; the nature of ideas, God himself, the soul, the beautiful and the good, and every intelligible essence, such as beauty itself, justice itself, equality itself, for we conceive each of these things as being one and as existing in itself."[25]

Since astronomical observations indicate inherent order and regular motion of the planetary bodies, Pythagoras concluded that the same numerical ratios that created harmony on the monochord must also apply to the universe.[26] Guthrie reminds us that the single string on the monochord instrument can be divided at any point, representing a continuum of infinite potential tones. But number is the means by which order is established to produce specific, rather than random, tones. The planets in their regular motions must create sounds similar to those Pythagoras discovered by moving the bridge on the monochord.[27] He called the sounds they accordingly produce "the music of the spheres."

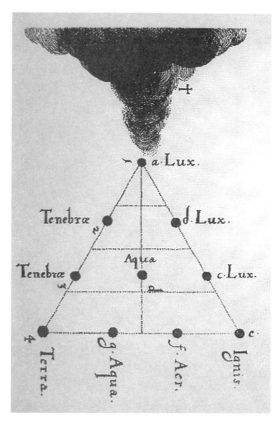

Fig. 7.12. Tetraktys showing four elements/humors at the base.
From Robert Fludd's *Philosophica Sacra* (1626).

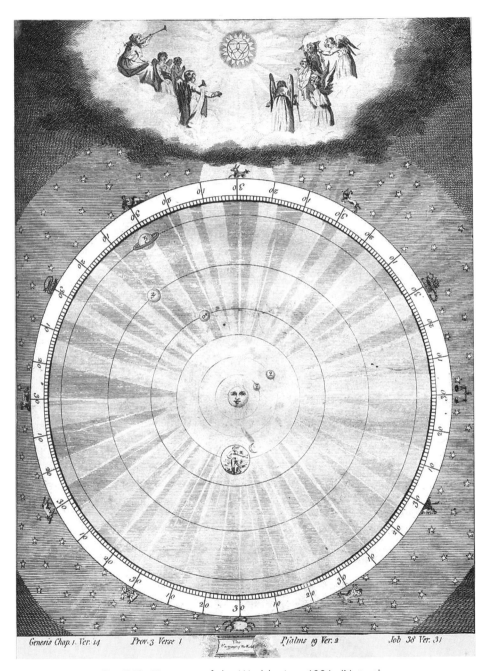

Fig. 7.13. Harmony of the World, circa 1806. (Note the astrological signs around the perimeter of the sphere.) By Ebenezer Sibly, from *A New and Complete Illustration of the Occult Sciences.*

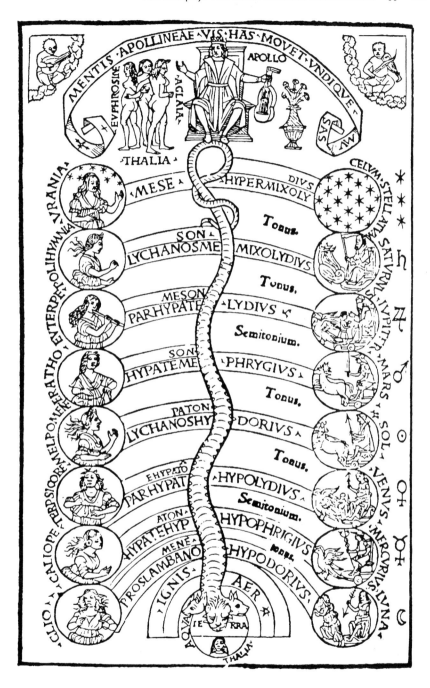

Fig. 7.14. Gafurius's *Practica musice* (1496): Renaissance engraving showing Apollo, the Muses, the planetary spheres and musical ratios. (Note the similarity to the serpentine spine discussed in chapter 6.)

MUSIC OF THE SPHERES

To fully understand the music of the spheres, we must come to an understanding of the phenomenon of harmonic overtones. As Guthrie explains: "A curious phenomenon occurs when a string is plucked. First, the string vibrates as a unit. Then, in two parts, then in three parts, four, and so on. As the string vibrates in smaller parts higher tones are produced, this being the so-called harmonic overtone series. While they are not as loud as the fundamental tone of the entire string vibrating, with practice the overtones can nonetheless be heard."[28]

On a stringed instrument such as a violin, harmonics are produced by lightly touching the string in these areas of division (half, third, and fourth), while plucking or bowing the string to produce the sound. If

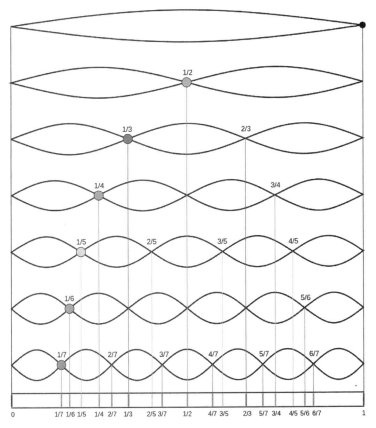

Fig. 7.15. Division of the string produces musical intervals and overtones.

the musician's left-hand finger is slightly off that precise ratio of the string, the harmonic won't sound clearly, or at all. In the same vein, if the musician's finger presses too much, rather than resting lightly on the string, the harmonic won't sound. One can see, then, that precise knowledge (based upon ratio and string division) is the technique that produces the subtle phenomenon of overtones.

The keyword here is *subtle*. Recalling the nature of manifestation through the elements as described by the tetraktys, subtle energy resides at the apex and denser energy toward the bottom. Resting lightly on the string produces subtle effects in the realm of vibration and sound. This phenomenon is important to understand when considering that acquired techniques are involved in both producing and hearing these subtle vibrations.

Pythagoras was known to have experienced and (according to his followers) was able to hear the higher harmonics produced by the planetary bodies in motion. Music harmony was dependent upon mathematical proportions, and Pythagoreans held that number was the means by which harmony and proportion kept everything in order in the cosmos. The music of the spheres describes metaphysical qualities of the mathematical relationships we find in number, geometry, music, and planetary orbits (astronomy). This order may also be extended to the periodic chart of all the atomic elements.

Manly Hall describes how Pythagoras established that music is an exact science.[29] He then applied his findings of harmonic intervals to other natural phenomena, extending them to the cosmos of planets and stars and to the classical elements. Later when organizing a table of the chemical elements according to their atomic weights, nineteenth-century chemist John Newlands (1837–1898) found repetition of distinctive properties in the progression of the elements according to harmonic ratio at every eighth element. Hall calls this finding "the law of octaves in chemistry." Modern chemists know it as the Periodic Table of the Elements for the periodic repetitions and correspondences found at every eighth element in the chart.

Hall described how the Pythagoreans came to consider themselves Canonics as they held that logic and mathematics, rather than sensory perception, must determine harmony.[30] Their position was in distinction from harmonic school musicians who based their principals of harmony on matters of instinctive feeling and taste. Pythagoras nonetheless recognized the deep effects of musical harmony on emotional feelings and the senses and attempted to mediate the mind-body connection in what he called "musical medicine."

In his early biography on Pythagoras, philosopher Porphyry (232–304), wrote: "He himself could hear the harmony of the Universe, and understood the music of the spheres, and the stars which move in concert with them, and which we cannot hear because of the limitations of our weak nature."[31]

Pythagorean philosophy stated that each body in the universe holds a specific tone and, by virtue of the fact that they moved, must be live entities. Contrary to the geocentric beliefs of his day, Pythagoras said that fire was the most important element and, as such, must be at the center of the cosmos, as would be the hearth of a home.

Hall contends it was natural for Pythagoras to divide the known cosmos into ten spheres represented by ten concentric circles.[32] The sacred number 10 represented the unity of everything and the sum of all components of the cosmos. These rings were conceptualized to begin with a globe of divine fire at the center, followed by the seven outward radiating planets, the Earth, and another obscure planet named Antichthon, which remained invisible due to its orbital path. It's interesting to note the "final" planet in our solar system remained invisible until the mid-twentieth century and was finally photographed in detail only in 2015 by a passing unmanned spacecraft.[33]

Hall surmised that the Antichthon may have referred to a mysterious eighth celestial sphere of the ancients, described as a dark planet that shared Earth's orbital path yet remained hidden from Earth on the other side of the sun. Perhaps this counter-earth theory influenced Pythagorean belief in the harmonization of opposites. More importantly, Pythagorean concepts emphasized that philosophical astronomy was a science of "realities" while physical astronomy was a science of shadows.[34] For now, at least, the reason behind this theory will also have to remain in the shadows.

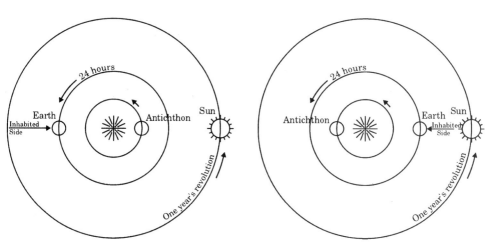

Fig. 7.16. Depiction of Antichthon (Counter-Earth) orbiting the central fire. The image (left) illustrates Earth at night, and the image (right) illustrates Earth in the daytime. From *Dante and the Early Astronomers* (1913), by M. A. Orr.

Another planet in which the Pythagoreans took great interest was Venus. Through its orbital relationship with Earth, Venus traces a geometric shape in the sky; this shape is known as the pentagram. The pentagram divides the 360-degree sphere into five sections equaling 72 degrees and creating the pentagon with dimensions divisible by phi.[35]

Pythagorean legacy provides at least two approaches to science and number; either with an eye to what quantitatively defines what is already known, or with an eye to discover the yet unknown.

To continue our discussion regarding phi's relationship to the cosmos, we return now to Plato who himself was a Pythagorean. Although differences in philosophy did exist between the two, Plato furthered Pythagorean geometric concepts that subsequently contributed to greater understandings in both astronomy and philosophy. The shapes written about in the Pythagorean fifth quarternary later became known as the platonic solids. Plato published information regarding the geometric forms of the four elements in Timeaus (circa 360 BCE).[36]

Author Kittie Ferguson brings to light a few of the philosophical differences between Plato and Pythagoras.[37] Basically, Pythagoreans believed that everything about the cosmos could ultimately be learned

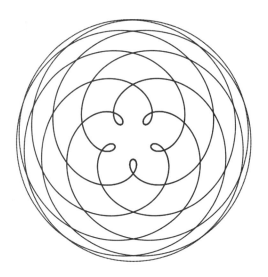

Fig. 7.17. The geocentric orbit of Venus.

through the process of discovering number—not quantitatively, but qualitatively. Pythagoreans believed that existential "Truth" lay deep beneath the surface like a vein of gold and that it would reveal itself to the initiate who practiced true science through the process of discovery.[38] However, they kept their knowledge in secret within "the brotherhood" to ensure that only the very well-disciplined initiate could practice it.

Plato, on the other hand, felt that the universe could never be known completely. The difference experienced was one of perception, with Pythagoreans focusing on knowing born from personal experience. Plato believed that a new method of education was necessary. Although he agreed that mathematics and geometry were part of the universal truth, they could not provide "the whole Truth" in its entirety.[39]

In the realm of music, these differences also surfaced. Plato believed that certain music could have deleterious effects on the soul and society. Pythagoreans used certain forms of music to heal and harmonize the psychic state, intent on unifying all areas of human life through the principles of harmony.[40] "The divine harmony can be grasped through the mind, yet can also be perceived through the senses . . . through praxis they may be felt in the soul, itself a harmonic entity."[41]

Wherever one stands regarding this subject, Plato's contributions are significant to our understanding of the cosmos.

PLATO'S DIALOGUES

As a Pythagorean, Plato was sworn to secrecy regarding certain reve-lations resulting from the study of number. Like Pythagoras himself, Egyptian priests had also trained Plato. In his writings, such as *Timaeus* and *The Republic,* he became adept at concealing deeper truths using mystical and mathematical metaphors.[42] Author Jamie James, in *The Music of the Spheres,* describes *Timaeus* as a cosmogonic rendition of Pythagorean mystical views regarding music, mathematics, and the cosmos.[43]

Professor of philosophy and comparative religion Scott Olsen states that in the *Timaeus* Plato presented philosophical conundrums that the reader must decipher, providing clues without ever divulging the answer.[44] In his dialogues, Plato carefully selected several interrelated problems that are very subtly posed. Taken together they point to the "great mystery of the Golden Section and its Reciprocal, none other than the Greater and Lesser of the Indefinite Dyad."[45]

Plato imparts to readers the notion "that continuous geometric pro-portion is the best of all bonds."[46] He proceeds to provide the "Lambda" Tetraktys (mentioned above regarding harmonic ratios), pointing the way to finding phi. In *The Republic,* he invites the reader to divide the line unevenly, referring to odd numbers as the "limited" world. As Olsen states, "In effect . . . telling us to generate a continuous geometric proportion between the whole and the parts with the simplest of all cuts, the Golden Cut."[47]

Plato provides the isosceles triangle, which when back-to-back creates the cube, and the equilateral triangle—the face of which constructs the tetrahedron, octahedron, and icosahedrons.[48] He delib-erately leaves out the triangle that would lead to the construction of the dodecahedron since that would reveal the golden section, as Hippasus had done. Instead, he challenges the reader to discover an even more beautiful triangle than the isosceles and equilateral.

With regard to the philosophical application of the golden mean, Olsen cites Plato's quote from his dialogue entitled *Statesman:* "'It is in this way, when they preserve the standard of the Mean that all their works are Good and Beautiful . . .The Greater and the Less are to be measured in relation, not only to one another . . . but also to the establishment of the standard of the Mean . . . This other comprises that which measures them in relation to the moderate, the fitting, the opportune, the needful, and all the other standards that are situated in the Mean between the Extremes.'"[49]

Now we've been indoctrinated to mathematics, literally and symbolically, as the mouthpiece for philosophical rendering. In the next chapter we look at how the golden ratio reveals itself in nature. Earth reveals itself in multiple and varied visual representations of "the mean between the extremes," or that which unites the parts with and within their wholes.

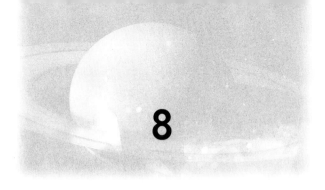

8

NATURE'S SPIN
A Sound Effect?

Big whorls have little whorls,
Which feed on their velocity;
And little whorls have lesser whorls,
And so on to viscosity.

LEWIS RICHARDSON (1881–1953)

We addressed the Pythagorean concepts of number, geometry, music, and astronomy in the previous chapter, and can now better understand Goethe's (1749–1832) statement "geometry is frozen music." We also explored the order implied by number, specifically the unifying aspect of phi, or Fibonacci's number, as expressed throughout nature—in space through geometry, in time through music, and in space-time through astronomy. Added to all these correspondences is the fact that everything great and small is dynamic and moving rather than stagnant—and where there is movement, vibration is generated. But the obverse is also true: Wherever vibration and sound occur, there is a corresponding impact on the environment. We may consider that as a plant grows its movement is not discernable to the naked eye. We can only see the results of its growth over time. We should also consider that sound is present whether or not the human ear can hear it.

In their revolutionary best-selling book, *The Secret Life of Plants,* authors Peter Tompkins and Christopher Bird reveal the hidden vibrational effects within the life of plants. They write: "What humans are able to perceive consciously with their limited senses is but a minute fraction of what vibrationally affects them . . . Efforts to prove that a given sonic vibration will affect plants or man may, far from resolving the interaction of music and life, be only unraveling a wondrously resonating tapestry of influences into its separate, unrelated threads."[1]

In this chapter, we explore how sound vibration is the likely force behind earthly phenomena, including the spiral patterns found from plant growth to weather, as we complete our tour of the four elements with earth and air. In the next, final chapter, we will examine how patterns of proportion and harmony that stem from phi and Fibonacci are also found in the human body—which behaves as a conductor for both cosmic and earthly frequencies. Seeing helps believing and we proceed with examples of how audible sound creates visible effects.

SOUND EFFECTS

To observe the effects of sound upon matter we may consider the work of German physicist and musician Ernst Chladni (1756–1827) and Swiss physician and scientist Hans Jenny (1904–1972). Chladni's contribution involved the discovery that sound waves generate certain patterns and shapes. His experiments used a violin bow drawn perpendicularly

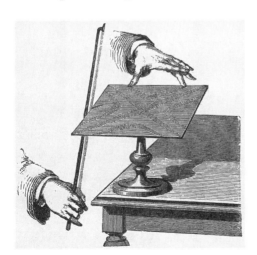

Fig. 8.1. Bow being applied to Chladni plate. From William Henry Stone (1879) *Elementary Lessons on Sound.*

across steel plates covered with sand or powder that produced different geometric designs when various tones were applied. The lower the frequency, the simpler the design; the higher the frequency, the more complex the design.

This breakthrough showed that sound visibly affects physical matter and produces patterns and shapes that are orderly and symmetrical.

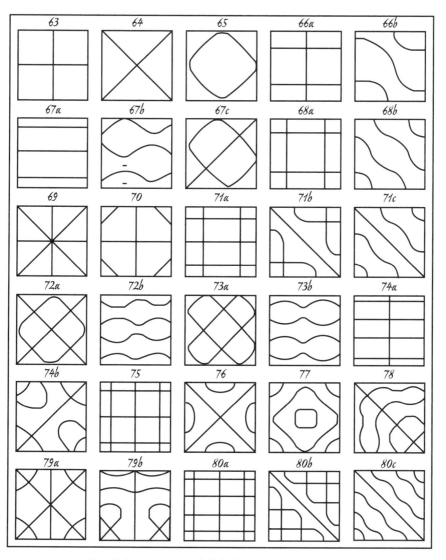

Fig. 8.2. Examples of Chladni acoustic patterns.
From E. F. F. Chladni, *Acoustics* (1802).

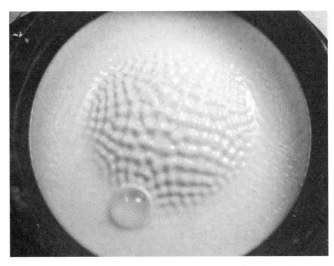

Fig. 8.3. Three-dimensional patterns created by sound applied to corn silk. Photograph by Collin Cunningham (CC BY-SA 3.0).

This discovery propelled the science of sound, and earned Chladni recognition as the "father of acoustics." What's also interesting is that his experiments showed that dry substances and particles (sand/powder) move away from the source of vibration to form the patterns.[2] Hans Jenny researched both dry and liquid substances, and determined that liquid moves toward vibration.

Instead of using the violin bow, Jenny invented something called a tonoscope, using crystal oscillators, that set plates vibrating, and his research has become known as *cymatics,* or the study of wave patterns (*cyma* means "wave").[3]

In acoustics, the terms *node* and *antinode* are used to describe minimum and maximum amplitudes (vibrations). With Chladni's experiments, dry particles were shown to move toward the nodes where minimum amplitude occurred. Jenny's discoveries showed that liquid would occupy the antinodes where maximum amplitude applied.[4] Furthermore, he discovered that sound's effects on liquid substances produced an anti-gravitational effect. As long as the vibration/tone was moving the substance, the plate could be tilted (inclined against gravity) and the shape could be maintained along the antinodal lines. When the vibration ceased, however, the substance would run (drain) down the plate![5]

Depending on frequency and amplitude, shapes would range from two-dimensional (close to the plate) to three-dimensional forms, influenced by the various characteristics of the materials used.[6]

In many of the experiments Jenny used plant spores (club moss) known as lycopodium powder. He found that when the tone was loud (large amplitude) the powder would be thrown up in fountains or even ejected. Yet by means of the stroboscope, which renders rapid phase sequences visible, he discovered that the patterns created by the vibration remained visible even in the dynamics of these eruptions.[7]

While the stroboscope was able to capture images, the tonoscope allowed Jenny to use the human voice when applying sound to different substances. He conducted experiments with people toning vowel sounds, and noticed how significant it was for the person to be able to see the effects of their spoken word. He realized that being able to see the effects of one's speech could be beneficial to those who could not hear as well as those who could. The tonoscope provided "visual speech" and enabled people to improve their communication skills and articulation.[8]

If vibration could be used in this way to benefit those unable to hear, it seems plausible (for this reason and others) that vibration could affect the silent world of plants as well. Even though plants cannot see or hear as people do, it doesn't necessarily mean they don't receive and respond to vibrations in their environment. On the contrary, living organisms seem to have a built-in communication system (as will be addressed a little later). Relevant from Jenny's research are the significant resemblances between the shapes and patterns we see in nature all around us and those generated from his acoustic research. Even phenomena resembling planetary motion, revolution, and rotation can be replicated through the application of sound.

Jenny recognized periodicity and rhythm as important underlying characteristics of vibrational influences upon nature as a whole, and on biological evolution and history.[9] Periodicity is the tendency for phenomena to recur in intervals, and rhythm is that which determines

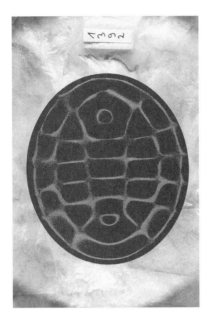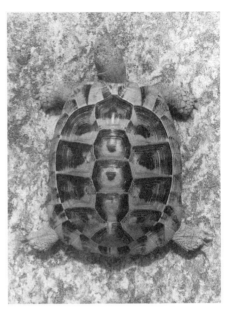

Fig. 8.4. Sound waves applied to sand creating tortoise image.
Photographs from *Water Sound Images* by Alexander Lauterwasser.
Copyright 2006 MACROmedia Publishing, Eliot, Maine.
www.cymaticsource.com. Used by permission.

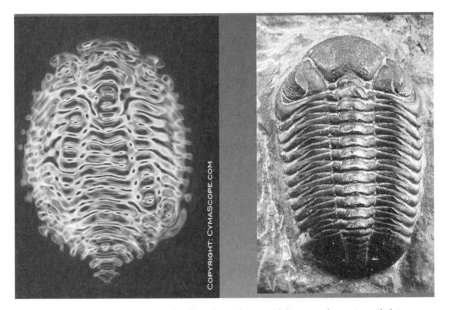

Fig 8.5. Sound waves applied to liquid resembling prehistoric trilobite.
Copyright Cymascope.com.

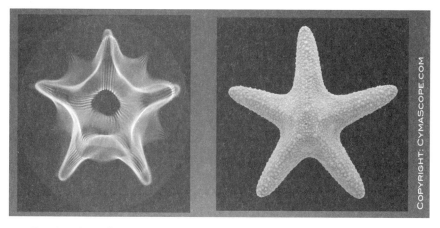

Fig. 8.6. Sound waves applied to liquid resembling prehistoric starfish. Copyright Cymascope.com.

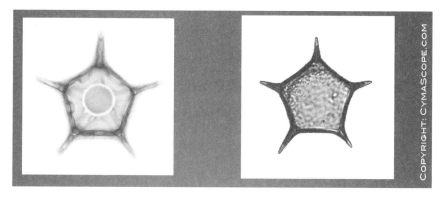

Fig. 8.7. Sound waves applied to liquid resembling fossilized diatom from sixty-five million years ago. Copyright Cymascope.com.

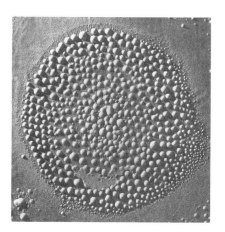

Fig. 8.8. Sound applied to lycopodium powder forms a number of round shapes, each rotating on its own axis and "orbiting" the central sphere. Photograph from *Cymatics: A Study of Wave Phenomena and Vibration* by Hans Jenny. Copyright 2001 MACROmedia Publishing, Eliot, Maine. www.cymaticsource.com. Used by permission.

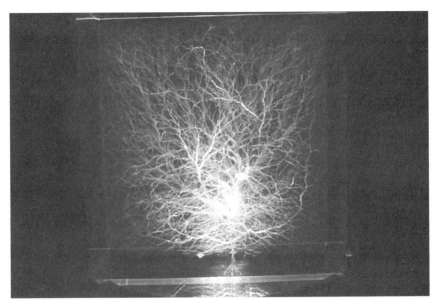

Fig. 8.9. Lichtenburg figure showing dendritic pattern.
Photo by Xylenol15 (CC BY 3.0).

the length (or timing) of that interval. For this study, he used German physicist Georg Christoph Lichtenberg's (1742–1799) experiments with electricity to draw attention to what caused the appearance of electrical, tree-like branching pathways, or fractal patterns. The figures produced branching dendritic formations similar to those found in plant leaves, branches, and roots, as well as the human body's circulatory, respiratory, lymphatic, biliary, exocrine, and nervous systems.

The point to note about these well-known Lichtenberg figures is that their morphology is characterized by the regularity of the discontinuities and thus by the tendency of their elements to be repetitive. They serve to draw attention to one of nature's most pervasive phenomena, which might be formulated as follows: Even without vibration in the narrow sense of the word, periodicity and seriality are disclosed in nature.[10]

It would appear that all elements contribute to creating natural and physical phenomena, and find pathways of expression through the principles of sound, vibration, rhythm, and interval. What we are really doing, then, is studying the morphology of vibration, or, in other words, drawing up an inventory of all the variety of forms in which it appears. We are not concerned with the play of the subjective mind but with the "objective play of nature," or with physics. Although it is always "the same," there is an enormous range of mutability in which each individual pattern nevertheless has its precise morphological characteristics. The resultants of harmonic vibrations are at all times so strictly law-ordered that it is possible to draw up a systematology of conditions. Nature produces this form only and no other. Nothing here is diffuse and indeterminate; everything presents itself in a precisely defined form.

The more one studies these things, the more one realizes that sound is the creative principle. It must be regarded as primordial. No single phenomenal category can be claimed as the original principle. We cannot say, in the beginning was number, or in the beginning was symmetry, etc. These are categorical properties which are implicit in what brings forth and what is brought forth. By using them in description we approach the heart of the matter. They are not themselves the creative power. This power is inherent in tone and in sound.[11]

This articulation of Jennys's reminds us that motion and morphology are constantly related. While there is an ordered manner in which the results of vibration are manifested, the manifestations themselves are subject to infinite variations and complexity. (There is a kind of feedback loop, which is discussed below.)

In *The World is Sound: Nada Brahama,* Joachim-Ernst Berendt describes sound as a phenomenon that, similar to the phi ratio, also dwells between the extremes: "It sounds in pulsars and planetary orbits, in the spin of electrons, in the quanta of atoms and the structure of molecules, in the microcosm and in the macrocosm. It also sounds in the sphere between these extremes, in the world in which we live."[12]

Berendt cautions that there is a difference between the statement "all is vibration" and a statement that the "world is sound." To Berendt, the difference comes down to one of perception. If we say the world is composed of vibration, the perception is one of random frequencies comingling without order. If we say that the world is composed of sound, the perception is one that acknowledges harmony and proportion implicit in the musical acoustic ordering of matter. In other words, both dissonance and consonance play vital roles in the natural self-regulating systems inherent in life. The organizing principle behind sound and the harmonizing effect implicit in it reconciles opposing forces.

THE SELF-REGULATING EARTH

Austrian–born American physicist Fritjof Capra, and Italian chemistry professor Pierre L. Luisi discuss this concept of reconciling opposing forces in *The Systems View of Life*. They posit that although nature can contain asymmetry at the molecular level, there is also a high degree of symmetry at the macroscopic level.[13] Asymmetry and symmetry coexist at both levels, however, asymmetry is more common to the microscopic world and symmetry more common to the macroscopic view. This seeming paradox may be taken as another example of how opposites give birth to each other and facilitate balance for one another: yin and yang; dark matter giving birth to light; and asymmetry in the molecular world giving rise to symmetry in the manifested realm. The authors discuss this principle within the context of James Lovelock's Gaia hypothesis, the idea that the Earth is a living, self-organizing, and self-regulating system.[14]

While working as a consultant for NASA in the 1960s, Lovelock noted the opportunity that allowed people to see the whole Earth suspended amidst the backdrop of dark space for the first time. He was struck by the stark beauty of this image. When the scientific community rejected his Gaia theory, Lovelock created a computer simulation called Daisyworld to demonstrate that the Earth self-regulates its temperature.

As a consequence of feedback loops among the planet's living organisms and their environments, as an example he showed how the growth of certain kinds of daisies would ebb and flow around the globe in response to the simulated temperature fluctuations on Earth for the purpose of helping to regulate those extremes.[15] The characteristics of sound in the form of pulsars, waves, periodicity, and rhythmic intervals are responsible for complex webs of communications. It seems reasonable to consider that they all contribute to, or actually comprise, the feedback mechanisms among life-forms.

Capra and Luisi discuss one of the questions physicists have been asking regarding how a universe exhibiting such symmetries across time and space still produces such a variety of form and function.[16] The answer, they propose, lies in the principle that some disturbance breaks up the symmetry, resulting in growth of diverse and complex patterns.[17] This concept may be related to the idea of rational and irrational numbers discussed in chapter 7. When enough duplication (symmetry) has occurred, irrational numbers introduce variety and "reboot/refresh" the system. When we look at number and geometry in plant life, known to botanists as phyllotaxis (from the same Greek root as *chloro-phyll,* but which could be called phi-llotaxis!), we see that interrupting a pattern of symmetry promotes growth, self-regulation, and variety. "The emergence of the Fibonacci sequence in phyllotaxis, and of the properties associated with it, can be traced back to specific dynamics of symmetry breaking in the growth pattern of the primordial (the first clumps of cells) at the tip of the plant's tiny shoot."[18]

SPIRALING INTO CONTROL

To include every example of spirals in the natural world would be impossible. It is important to distinguish other spirals from the golden spiral, and our focus will remain mostly on the latter. In this way, we can continue to see it in nature wherever number, geometry, music, and astronomy find expression. There is a certain spiral (see fig. 8.10) named after Greek mathematician Archimedes (circa 287–212 BCE), in which growth or propagation occurs at a fixed rate. The helix pattern is a three-dimensional version of this spiral.[19] Logarithmic spirals, also known as equiangular spirals, so named by René Descartes in the seventeenth century, contain properties of self-reproduction, or propagation. They comprise a family of spirals whose growth occurs at a constant angle.[20] The golden spiral (fig. 8.11) belongs in this family of spirals, yet also has a unique association with the Fibonacci number sequence.

Capra and Luisi state:

The logarithmic spiral has several unique properties that help us understand why it appears so frequently in nature. It is defined mathematically as a curve that is magnified by the same factor (known as its growth rate) in successive turns through a constant angle around its origin (or "pole"). In other words, the spiral's radius (a straight line between the pole and a point on the curve) increases in geometric progression with each turn. Different growth rates will produce different geometric progressions, and hence different logarithmic spirals. The golden spiral is a particular logarithmic spiral that grows by a factor of φ (the golden ratio) for every quarter turn.[21]

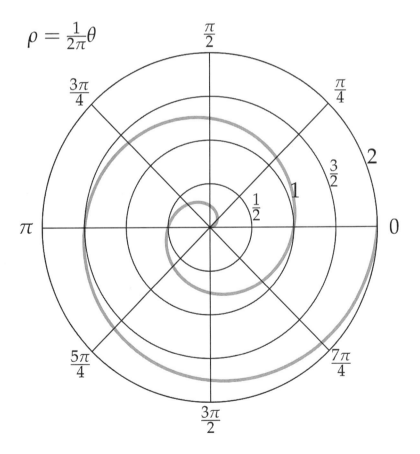

$$\rho = \frac{1}{2\pi}\theta$$

Fig. 8.10. Archimedes spiral. By Guillaume Jacquenot (CC BY-SA 3.0).

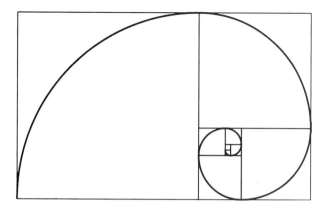

Fig. 8.11. Golden spiral.

Numerous examples of the golden spiral exist in nature, however; the sunflower, pinecone, and pineapple have held particular fascination among biologists and botanists for centuries.[22] In figure 8.12 we see an actual sunflower, and figure 8.13 describes the Fibonacci growth sequence.

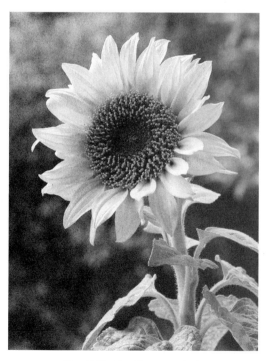

Fig. 8.12. Sunflower spiral.

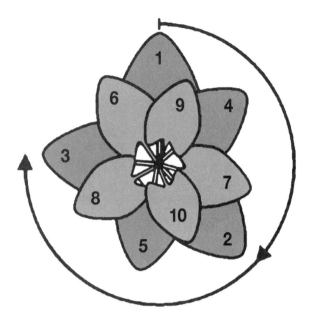

Fig. 8.13. The angle between successive florets in some flowers is the golden angle. By Wolfgangbeyer (CC BY-SA 3.0).

As we discussed earlier in chapter 6, the pinecone has held spiritual significance for centuries due to its resemblance to the pineal gland. We also see references to the dandelion in esoteric art. Perhaps a more compelling reason for this fascination is due to the relationship the pinecone and dandelion have to the golden spiral.

It was believed that plants follow this particular spiral growth pattern to optimize the process of photosynthesis. Now biologists know that the same growth pattern exists in saltwater algae, constantly moved by water currents, as well as other life-forms that do not require light. Given the enormous variety of forms found in the plant kingdom, the authors emphasize how the Fibonacci spiral is found so abundantly.[23] "For example, if we count the number of clockwise or counterclockwise spirals in a sunflower or in a pineapple, then usually we will find two successive Fibonacci numbers . . . This is true even in instances where we would hardly expect them, such as in the flower heads . . . of dandelions. After all the sailing dandelions seeds

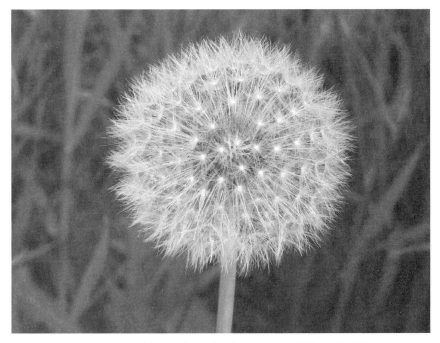

Fig. 8.14. Dandelion. Photo by Greg Hume (CC BY-SA 3.0).

have been dispersed, a Fibonacci spiral pattern . . . can be seen."[24]

If we consider Lovelock's Gaia hypothesis that the Earth has a built-in self-regulating mechanism, perhaps it has something to do with the Fibonacci (or golden) spiral. In *The Glorious Golden Ratio,* Posamentier and Lehmann offer support for Capra and Luisi's subsequent explanation that it is precisely the pressure of an opposing force that provides the means by which "regulation" occurs, breaking up the symmetry at the primordial tip to produce a new shoot.[25]

UNDER PRESSURE

Mathematician Dr. J. N. Ridley developed a simulation model based on Swiss botanist Simon Schwendener's (1829–1919) "contact-pressure hypothesis" and Johannes Kepler's research on the mechanical forces that lead to specific organic forms and patterns.[26] In this model, Ridley "explained that the rhombic form of pomegranate seeds is due to the pressure contact on the seeds during growth. As a result of these pressure forces, tightly packed rhombic seed structures are generated . . . The compact packing of the leaf primordial makes the hypothesis of pressure-force related forms in the early development stages plausible."[27]

Ridley's algorithm includes three stages: 1) generation of the new primordium, 2) interaction of the primordial, and 3) expansion of the primordial.[28] These stages can be taken to describe in miniature what happens in space when new stars and galaxies are born. The compaction of matter creates heat that builds to maximum radiation until new "life" and expansion burst open, creating the spiral. Ridley's simulation model showed that for a majority of areas, the spiral pattern generated was precisely the one we find most often in nature—the golden spiral: "For the sunflower, this is with a frequency of 82 percent Fibonacci spirals and 14 percent Lucas spirals."[29]

Thus, as Capra and Luisi state, the growth pattern of sunflower seeds features two sets of interpenetrating spirals, one clockwise and the other counterclockwise.[30] They also state that the number of spirals typically turns out to be two consecutive Fibonacci numbers, generated by the golden angle as is found in helical phyllotaxis. "In 1979, biophysicist Helmut Vogel created a mathematical model representing the growth patterns of the corresponding primordia and was able to show that only the golden angle produces a tight packing of the seed head. Even a slight change of the angle causes the pattern to break up into a single family of spirals with gaps between the seeds."[31]

It would seem, then, that the contraction inherent in "phi-llotaxis" is what helps create the particular growth pattern so prevalent in nature. More importantly, perhaps, is that it facilitates the maintenance and equilibrium required for sustaining and propagating life.

Tompkins and Bird referred to the research of Donald Hatch Andrews (1898–1980), who had been a longtime chemistry professor at Johns Hopkins University, and in 1967 authored *The Symphony of Life*.[32] Andrews's book invited the reader on an imaginary journey inside the world of plants. He remained a proponent of the idea that sound vibration also lay at the heart of all atomic structures, and believed that inside the atom vibrated tones of great musical complexity that included dissonance.[33]

Tompkins and Bird also described the beliefs of English composer and theosophist Cyril Meir Scott that a function of dissonant music was to break up thought forms that create stagnation among whole countries and peoples—similar to the way in which disturbances break up symmetry, resulting in growth of more diverse and complex patterns.[34] It may also be seen as similar to the way in which irrational numbers break up duplication, producing infinite variety.

Tompkins and Bird also refer to the work of Hans Kayser (1891–1964) in *Harmonia Plantarum* (1943). Kayser wrote about the musical octaves and intervals related to plant growth, particularly the correspondence of octaves to the shapes of plants. "Kayser observed that if one projects all tones within the space of one octave—in the same manner that the astronomer and astrologer Johannes Kepler worked out in his Harmonica Mundi for the solar planetary system—and sketches their angles in a specific way, one obtains the prototype of leaf form. The interval of the octave, the basis for music making and indeed all sensation, thus contains within itself the form of the leaf."[35]

Having had a look at Earth's plant life we now turn our attention to the sky. Looking up, we continue with the idea that there is a burst of energy (which may be likened to plant primordia) at the level of the birth of stars that is generated by sound. Jenny reminds us that oscillations are ever present in nature and, consequently, we should expect to find periodic, rhythmic, and cyclic phenomena constantly.[36] He believed that everything in our environment could be explained in terms of sound waves (cymatics), including atmospheric phenomena.

Hardly ever do we look at the sky by day without seeing periodic elements. Even in a cloudless sky the upward and downward movement of spheres of haze can be observed. No sooner are filaments of clouds spun out of the blue sky than an endless pageant of changing forms begins . . . But if we look carefully, we shall see that at one end it is continually dissolving, while at the other end it is continually forming again. Thus it is not a fixed, unchanging object that we are looking at, but rather a process. What persists is the activity, as it were, of the "cloud" . . . And if we span our vision to take in ever more extensive nexus of atmospheric phenomena, we become aware of vast formations . . . The tendency to repetition is found not only on the regional, but also the supraregional scale . . . However small or large our field of vision, we find waves, interpenetrating waves, circulations, pulsations, cyclic layers, serial fronts, periodic creation and extinction, rhythmic morphology . . . Whether we are following the mode of origin of a single raindrop or looking down upon the global pattern of vortices through the eyes of the astronauts, it is always this vision of interwoven phenomena that we see, dominated by periodicity and rhythmicity.[37]

PHI IN THE SKY

The spirals that form in Earth's atmosphere are dependent on fluctuations in temperature and on differences in surface terrain that affect temperature. There can be anything from thermal waves, to hurricanes, to the violent vortices of tornados. In a thermal, the sunny side of the terrain absorbs heat so that the air above is warmed there, while air above the shadowed terrain remains cooler. Since buildings absorb heat, they can also create similar effects. The differences in temperature create convective currents causing the air to circulate. As cold and warm fronts meet, this process intensifies; such air currents can ultimately create the extreme spirals of hurricanes.[38] (This temperature flux and interaction mirrors that said of the four element characteristics: hot, cold, moist, dry, the mixing of which causes an impact on the environment, whether human body, earth, or atmosphere.)

When interrupted (like the interruption of symmetrical patterns in plant growth) by objects on the Earth's surface such as islands, mountains, or even buildings, airstreams and cloud currents form interesting patterns. Called *cloud streets,* they form a series of spheres and vortices (see fig. 8.15).

In certain instances, one can observe a relationship between storm formation and the golden spiral, such as the case of Hurricane Sandy in October 2012 (see fig. 8.16).

Atmospheric spirals also seem to function as "roads in the air" that

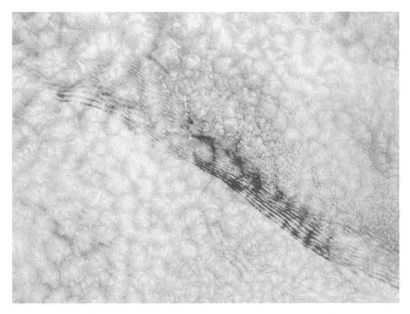

Fig. 8.15. Cloud streets and von Karman vortices, Greenland Sea.
Photo credit, NASA.

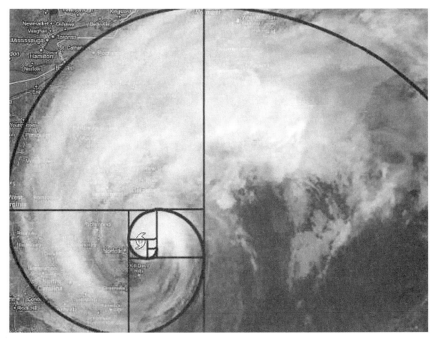

Fig. 8.16. Hurricane Sandy Fibonacci spiral. Photo credit, NASA.

birds follow to achieve a goal or reach their destination. In *The Golden Ratio*, Mario Livio points out that the peregrine falcon follows air currents that flow in a logarithmic spiral.[39] This particular falcon is one of the fastest birds, plummeting up to two hundred miles per hour toward its intended target. Their eye placement is bilateral rather than frontal, and they would have to tilt their heads at a 40-degree angle if they were to follow a straight-line path, which would have the effect of slowing them down considerably. Following the path of the spiral allows them to optimize use of their powerful vision as well as their speed.[40]

Aerospace engineer Jeff Scott says that watching birds is one of the best methods scientists have of identifying thermal currents. Ironically, he states that birds often "do the same thing," that is, watch pilots to determine the location of these currents. When a pilot discovers a thermal to utilize he or she may soon find birds joining the flight.[41]

The currents and spirals within Earth's atmosphere represent another example of the constant movement between expansion and diminution we find at every level of nature. Depending on the type of manifestation, we may find other forms. Author of several books on sacred geometry, Karen French says: "Circles establish time, squares design space and triangles are the basis of Being. The Trinity of simple, yet profoundly important, geometric shapes together generate an impenetrable mesh; a Matrix of Space-Time-Being permeating reality on every scale imagineable."[42]

We now turn our attention to a much larger cycle, where we see how the rhythm and periodicity of planets play a role in the matrix of space-time.

PLANETARY PERIODICITY

Although the space above Earth's atmosphere is not breathable "air," there is still relevance in exploring the connection we see between increasingly larger cycles and the Fibonacci number.[43] Olsen writes that the golden ratio is found abundantly in our solar system, stating that the mean orbits of Mercury, Jupiter, and Saturn in relationship to Earth all form geometric shapes that are divisible by phi with 99.99 percent accuracy. For example, he states that "the relative mean orbits of Earth and Mercury are given by ϕ^2: 1, or a pentagram, to 99 percent accuracy."[44]

In the previous chapter we briefly mentioned the pentagram Venus draws in its orbit around the Earth. Significant about this relationship is that it has the Fibonacci numbers 13, 8, and 5. Eight Earth years "transpose" to 13 Venus years, and Venus's 8-year path around the sun (from Earth's perspective) draws the 5-pointed pentagram in the sky.[45] As both the morning and the evening star (inside the Earth's own orbit around the sun, and always "close" to it as seen in the sky at dawn and dusk) her appearances to the ancients became associated with opposing forces. However, the astrological association for Venus's archetype is one of harmonizing the opposites.

Here again we are reminded that opposing forces are found all around us, but can be perceived as a way to maintain equilibrium. Whether dissonance or consonance, asymmetry or symmetry, nature reveals itself through the dance of opposites on every scale.

Sound and vibration may be found from the barely discernable movements in plant growth to the instantaneous flashes of lightning in Lichtenberg's figures, to the spherical motions of the clouds in the atmosphere, to the geometric proportions drawn by planets in our sky. Sound vibration may be the creative "first cause," and also the organizing principle maintaining harmony and balance. In the next, final, chapter we continue to explore these principles while considering the human anatomy as a conduit between earth and cosmos. We will also discover how sound can restore healing and balance, including an application through the system of Chinese medicine.

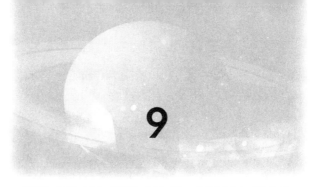

9

THE FUTURE AWAITS
OUR RETURN

When you have been compelled by circumstances to be disturbed in any manner, quickly return to yourself, and do not continue out of tune longer than the compulsion lasts. You will have increasing control over your own harmony by continually returning to it.

MARCUS AURELIUS (CIRCA 161–180)

Throughout this book we have looked at patterns and correspondences we find from our ancient past to determine how they express themselves in the four elements: earth, air, fire, and water. Now we look at human anatomy with the purpose of connecting these concepts to medicine. True health involves relationship with the whole, and relationship always involves change. The elements never remain in their current states for long, but are continually combining, recombining, and interacting to form other substances. Another aspect of healing has to do with "re-membering," calling back parts of ourselves that have been lost or abandoned in some way, creating tension for the purpose of being integrated with the whole.

In *Sacred Science*, Schwaller de Lubicz states that harmony is a cosmic law from which all order in the physical world is derived, and all forms come into being. In *Cosmic Octave* Hans Cousto creatively defines the transposition of planetary tones into frequencies accessible to human hearing. Joachim-Ernst Berendt reminds us that corrective hearing, those minor micro adjustments that allow us to perceive music, can be found everywhere in nature, including in plants, animals, human anatomy, and the cosmos. In *Acutonics From Galaxies To Cells,* Carey, et al. have compiled an anthology of living wisdom regarding the relationship between the cosmos and humanity with examples of applied planetary harmonic medicine.

Sound is an effective means by which we can restore harmony to the whole. As we saw in the last chapter, sound arranges and rearranges forms according to the principles of harmony. By recognizing where we have gone out of balance (into polarity stagnation), we can use sound to support greater awareness of the whole, and leverage self-regulating capacity at the micro and macro levels to restore balance.

Proceeding with the premise that geometry can be perceived as "frozen music," we look at how the application of astrological principles can assist in the process of "returning to self" through the medium of sound. When certain mathematical relationships and ratios in the natal chart become "frozen" geometric "attitudes"—causing stagnation and dissonance—sound can facilitate the movement toward harmony. In continuity with the previous chapters regarding the recurrence of phi in nature and the cosmos, we begin by looking at where we find geometry and proportion in human form.

GEOMETRY AND PROPORTION IN ANATOMY

As we observe the golden proportion, or Fibonacci sequence, and geometry in the natural world, we also find them in human anatomy. Schwaller de Lubicz states that when the golden proportion is expressed in physical form, it first requires division into two equal (symmetrical) parts.[1] The example he gives is that of a newborn baby's height, which is divided equally at the navel. During childhood the lower body grows at a more rapid pace than do the head and upper body, and as the individual matures, growth follows the phi ratio. As an adult, the navel of the individual no longer divides the body in equal halves, but rather in proportion to the golden mean.[2]

Put another way, the navel comes to divide the whole body as the eyebrow divides the whole face.[3] Schneider states that phi divides the distance from the nose to the base of the neck, from the neck to the armpit, from armpit to navel, from navel to the tip of the fingers (while arms are pointing to the ground), and from the fingertips to the soles of the feet.[4] Thus, the body is divided seven times by the golden mean.[5]

History's prototypical legendary artist, scientist, and Renaissance man was also fascinated by phi, and contributed some of science and medicine's most accurate and precise information on anatomy, geometry, and proportion. Leonardo da Vinci's legacy is so prolific we can barely scratch the surface of it, however, what pertains to anatomical geometry and proportion is relevant to this discussion.

THE LEGACY OF LEONARDO

Man is the measure of all things.
PROTAGORAS (CIRCA 490–420 BCE)

In *Learning from Leonardo*, Fritjof Capra outlines the extent to which Leonardo da Vinci (1452–1519) left clues to the many natural connections linking today's artificially separated natural sciences: anatomy, botany, ecology, geology, and physics.[6] In *Vitruvian Man* (circa 1490), da Vinci captures the geometric proportions found in human anatomy (microcosm), first illustrated by Roman architect Vitruvius (80 BCE–15 BCE) that mirror the macrocosm. Of particular interest were the square, the circle, and the golden section.[7]

Whereas Vitruvius had separated descriptions of the body within a circle from that of the body within a square, Leonardo unified them (see fig. 9.1). Inscribed in the figure of man within the circle is: if the legs are open to the point at which height is decreased by 1/14, and the arms are raised so that the middle fingers align with the crown of the head, then the navel will be the center of arm and leg extremities and the space between the legs will form an equilateral triangle.[8]

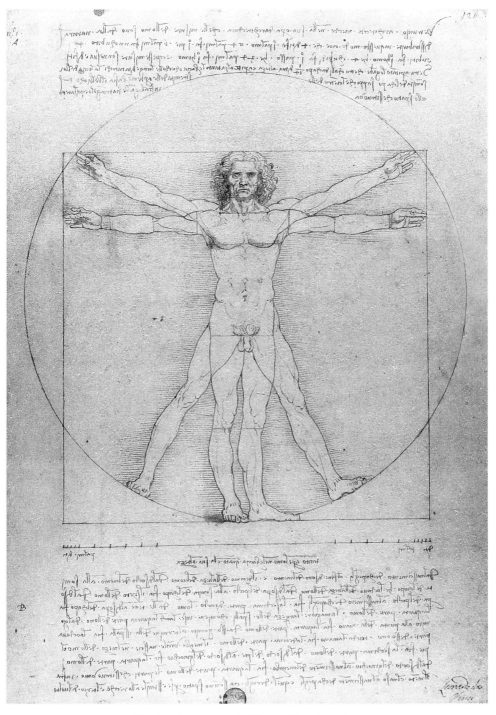

Fig. 9.1. Leonardo da Vinci's *Vitruvian Man*.

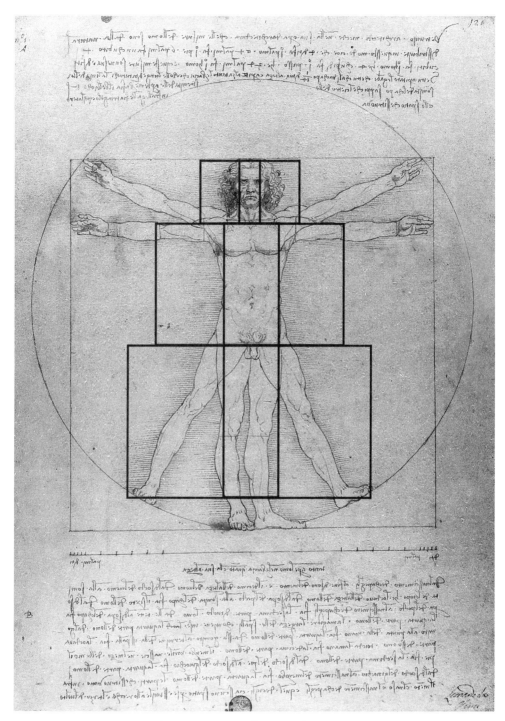

Fig. 9.2. *Vitruvian Man* showing phi proportions.

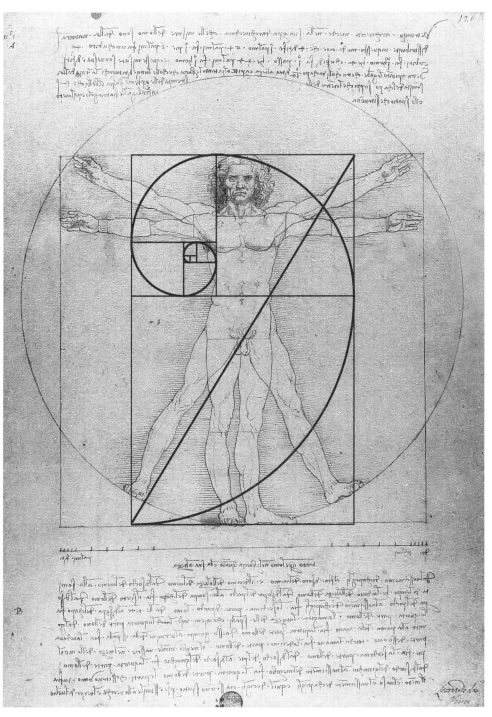

Fig. 9.3. *Vitruvian Man* with golden spiral.

FIBONACCI SPIRAL

Inscribed in the figure of man within the square is the understanding that the outstretched arm span will equal a man's height (see fig. 9.3). The measurement from the roots of the hair (hairline, scalp) to the bottom of the chin is 1/10 of a man's height. From the crown of the head to the bottom of the chin is 1/6 of the man; the maximum width of the shoulders equals 1/4 of the height, and "the complete hand is the tenth part of the man."[9]

Leonardo's work stood apart from artists who preceded him in that he realized that a concentric rendition of the circle and square would unnaturally distort the body. Instead, he chose the navel as the center of the figure in the circle, and the pubic bone as the center of the figure in the square. This distinction is interesting when placed in the context of Schwaller de Lubicz and Schneider who show human growth obeys the phi ratio wherein the navel no longer represents the center. Also interesting is that the three-dimensional sphere (two-dimensional circle) represents spirit, and a state to which the newborn baby would be closest, whereas, an adult has been fully indoctrinated into the material realm (square), and therefore a different center point would apply. Leonardo also emphasized mathematical precision as a constant without sacrificing the presence of change and transformation. His major contribution to science is characterized by the investigation of forms that included both qualitative and quantitative dimensions, reflecting the opposites, and always seeking to synthesize them to the whole.[10]

HARMONY, SYNTHESIS, AND THE COSMIC WHOLE

Leonardo's principle medical consultant was Modino de Luzzi (circa 1270–1326), a professor at Bologna who emphasized that successful anatomical dissection of body parts depended upon keeping a whole-body perspective.[11] Through their association, Leonardo came to learn about Avicenna's *Canon of Medicine* and Galen's humoral medicine (see chapter 2). Leonardo took from their teachings what worked, dismissing what didn't correlate with his own experience.[12] Throughout his life, Leonardo remained focused on proving that geometric division and variation in the body could be integrated into a harmonious whole. Scientist and historian Domenico Laurenza states: "He attempts systematically to realize representations that reconstitute the extreme variety and variability of the individual anatomical parts (displayed in the course of the dissections) into a harmonious composition . . . Around 1506–1508, he creates anatomical representations which not only show the organs as an ensemble, in their reciprocal relationships, but also emphasize the symmetry of some of them."[13]

Leonardo's goal to show harmony and synthesis in anatomy found expression and flourished during the first half of the sixteenth century. But by mid-century, the shift to analyzing anatomical dissections, separate from the composite whole, had taken place. Just a quarter-century following Leonardo's death (1543), Flemish anatomist Andreas Vesalius came to prominence with his *Fabrica,* an extensive volume with over two hundred illustrations of regional anatomical dissections of humans and animals.[14]

Capra writes that Leonardo repeatedly emphasized the virtues of *cognizione integrale* (integral knowledge), while denouncing the analytical perspective of isolating parts as *cosa mostruosa* (monstrous thing) in anatomical studies.[15] Thus, Leonardo anticipated the reductionist future directions of science, which would separate and isolate the pieces and parts from the whole in a self-circumscribed quest that achieved only a limited understanding of nature.

THE WHOLE CONTINUUM

When addressing the relations of microcosm (anatomy and its internal system) with macrocosm (expansion to infinity) Leonardo also mentions pyramidal architectural structure. "All natural powers . . . are to be called pyramidal inasmuch as they have degrees in continuous proportion toward their diminution as toward their increase."[16]

Leonardo believed that the pyramid, a tetrahedron as explained earlier, provides a symbolic link connecting micro to macro transformation and function.[17] As has been stated throughout this book, pyramidal structures held significance throughout antiquity, particularly with regard to the fire element and light absorption. Thus, Leonardo's belief also supports Edward Bynum, who discusses the light-absorbing function of melanin in light of its tetrahedral shape.[18]

Leonardo's legacy regarding harmony and synthesis of all parts within the whole was not limited to human anatomy. He also included theories involving the body's organ system as analogous to how Earth sustains life within the context of our solar system.[19] Capra explains that one of Leonardo's early theories compared the flow of blood in humans to that of water flow on Earth, and the flow of sap in plants, believing each process to be maintained by the heat of the sun. He used the term *humor* to describe vital fluids, and believed the sun's heat raised these fluids inside the human body as it does with the Earth. Inasmuch as Earth's water nourishes vegetation, and sap from the vegetation nourishes "plant tissues," human blood nourishes the organs and tissues in the body.[20]

Leonardo's idea that the heart's function in the body is analogous to that of the sun in the solar system was consistent with ancient philosophy, based principally upon Hermeticism, which as we know, is the sacred law handed down through the teachings of Hermes Trismegistus (also Egyptian god Thoth), discussed in chapter 2. The sun is responsible for providing life to the whole universe, and to the animals and plants of the Earth. The heart's function of pumping blood throughout the body to nourish cells and tissues is as crucial to its survival as are the rays of the sun to life on Earth.

HERMETIC POTENTIAL
IN HUMAN BEINGS

Freke and Gandy provide a translation of *The Hermetica,* in which Hermes describes the sun as an image of the Creator, which nourishes all vegetation, animals, and plants in the same way the supreme Creator gives life to the whole universe.[21]

In another excerpt Hermes describes creation hierarchy (with the Cosmos being made in the image of the Creator and the sun and planets following) providing light and life on Earth. Even while describing the sun as "the greatest god in the heavens," he emphasizes that it and all things in creation fall under the purview of the One who keeps everything in order, even that which appears to be "out of measure" (out of sync): "The sun is the greatest god in the heavens . . . Yet, this mighty god humbly submits to have smaller stars circle above him . . . even disorder is subject to the Master who has yet to impose order upon it."[22]

Where structure and geometry are concerned, mathematician, researcher, and author Michael S. Schneider supports the "As above, so below" Hermetic principle, stating it is a law that extends to the physical realm and human anatomy.

> We contain smaller similar structures and we are part of, and models of, larger structures of the cosmos . . . Thus the human body itself models greater self-replicating wholes. Its expanding φ proportion recurs in the larger structure of the solar system, in the distances of the planets from the sun and each other. Here the additive Fibonacci process is at work: the distance from the sun to Mercury plus Mercury's distance to Venus equals the distance between Venus and Earth . . . The φ ratio is most clearly defined by the planets nearest the sun, but the ideal gradually breaks down toward the outer planets . . . In this way the solar system is a great body, perhaps a form of life we don't recognize as such.[23]

In a passage from *The Hermetica,* Hermes is credited with describing how the body is constructed by the "power of the Zodiac" (part of the hierarchy and electromagnetic structure affecting human anatomy discussed in chapter 5).

> The human body is an earthly temple constructed by the power of the Zodiac, which makes myriad forms from simple archetypes. There are twelve signs of the Zodiac and the forms they produce fall into

twelve divisions. They are, however, inseparably united in their action. Nature makes the human body so that its constitution resonates with the patterns of the stars, in such a way that they mutually affect one another. When we are born . . . these particular powers that change according to the rotation of the planets make their way in through the body, and mould the shape of our souls. They penetrate our nerves and marrow, veins and arteries, even our innermost organs.[24]

CHINA'S CONNECTION TO HERMETICISM, HOROSCOPES, AND HUMAN CARTOGRAPHY

In his book *China's Cosmological Prehistory,* Laird Scranton draws parallels between the ancient cultures of (southern) Africa, Egypt, India, and Asia, some of which were discussed in chapter 2, pointing out the similarities in meaning that certain symbols came to have. For instance, he explains that owls symbolized knowledge, elephants came to mean abundance, and the serpent—originally revered in all cultures—eventually took on an evil connotation.[25]

He also shares what he considers to be a curious connection between Egypt and China having to do with the two cultures choosing similar measurements of time (albeit based on planetary movements): the 360-day year, 30-day month, 10-day week, 24-hour day, and 60-minute hour.[26]

This holds significance where the Western astrology chart is concerned. Up to this point, our focus on Chinese medicine has had more to do with the elements. However, we will now address the meridian correspondence to the horoscope.

In the horoscope chart, we have a 360° circle that has the sun following a 30° movement through one month that is assigned to a zodiac sign; each 30°sign is divided into three decants of 10°. Within a twenty-hour day, we have zodiac signs changing every two hours on the eastern horizon, which holds significance for the birth-time of an individual; twenty-four hours divided by two equals twelve signs in the zodiac circle. Coincidentally, there are twelve "regular" meridians in Chinese medicine, which also follow the circadian clock so that each meridian is assigned two hours within a given day. Finally, we have the degrees and minutes of the zodiac signs within the horoscope chart corresponding to the sixty-minute hour.

Ancient cultures from both the east and west credited their knowledge to the influence of celestial beings, and by whatever means it came to be transferred from culture to culture around the globe, the Chinese were able to develop a profound medical system with sophisticated mapping of meridian lines that facilitate energy movement in the body. The Chinese have always maintained that this cartography is one that reflects the constellations in the heavens, thus mirroring the Hermetic principle "As above, so below."

To detail the implications of a human grid-work (lattice, matrix, hologram) that syncs up with the macrocosmic grid-work is beyond the bounds of our current discussion. However, we can see in esoteric works such as *The Book of Knowledge: The Keys of Enoch* by J. J. Hurtak, that these meridian lines may hold the key to tapping into an infinite source of healing.[27]

There is at work within all biological systems a path of interchangeability to standardize unique vibratory levels. Our galactic body of creation controls its renewing functions through meridian axiatonal lines which are the equivalent of acupuncture lines that can connect with resonating star systems. These axiatonal lines are not limited to a physical body or a biological creation, but are open-ended and can connect the body vehicle with axiatonal lines that emanate from the various star populations and exist as chemical code mechanisms. When Man can discover the connection between this life space and the axiatonal grids controlling the body through endless cell division, Man will have a new superscience known as medical astronomy.[28]

Interchangeability, unlimited access to renewing faculties, and open-endedness are concepts that deserve our consideration. Change itself is a governing principle of the universe that occurs in an orderly, measured, rhythmic way through time (as we perceive it). The fundamental laws of nature, however, are taken to be "changeless," because they are permanent, and the means by which we measure those cycles remains unchanging—at least at this point in our history. This view is what the ancients considered to be the spiraling, rotating order of the universe, the expansion of which seems to occur proportionately to the golden mean, which creates infinitely as it reconciles all to the One.

Hermetic initiates believed that a Supreme Deity intended and actuated order and harmony throughout Creation. In the process of doing so, it imprinted its image on all matter from the greater to the lesser cycles, leaving its corresponding signature on planetary bodies in our solar system, the Earth, and life-forms on Earth. This has been stated when addressing the hierarchy of the heavens from the unmanifested to the manifested realms.[29]

During the sixteenth century, physician, botanist, and astrologer, Paracelsus, made this doctrine of signatures and concept of correspondences better known. Christian mystic and theologian Jacob Boehme spread the influential concept of the "doctrine of signatures" in *The Signature of All Things* (1621), describing how the Creator marks all living creatures, including plants, animals, and stones with a signature corresponding to that of the planets and the healing properties each therein.[30]

THE DOCTRINE OF SIGNATURES

In *The Doctrine of Signatures,* the late Scott Buchanan, a philosopher and author who had a particular interest in medical science, describes the doctrine:

> [N]ature holds within its patterns certain discoverable uniformities . . . it says that things are governed by laws. Finally it says that there are always empirical ways of discovering these uniformities and laws . . . these ways . . . had a long history before the middle ages. . . . best expressed in the myth that now goes by the name, the doctrine of signatures. This myth says that when God created man and made him subject to ills and misfortunes He also created stones, plants,

animals, and other human beings and marked them with characteristic marks to be recognized and used as remedies. He gave man the ability to read these signatures both in himself and in natural objects and to interpret them for the good of his soul and body.[31]

The idea of anthropomorphism imbuing all life-forms with an image of man, which in turn is an "image of the Divine," is discounted by modern science but proves to be useful. If the nature of science involves exploring mystery for the purpose of explaining it, it must first understand the source of that mystery. Our current medical model is completely out of sync with those who are by nature "spiritual," and to whom the notion of separating parts in exclusion from the composite body is equally absurd. Knowing the operations of energy, especially in terms of the morphing process of the four elements, we must consider the metaphysical properties of form, particularly that of the human body.

When addressing the relevancy of anthropomorphism, Buchanan explained that the human body as well as man's relationship to his environment is the inescapable reality that must be the focus and source of study.[32] He addressed the issue incumbent upon medical science to study the mysteries of metaphysics even when inconvenient. "The metaphysics of form and matter supplies a system of double-entry book-keeping for any science, and although a science such as chemistry or physics may dodge the necessity, it seems that medicine which is man's study of man should not take chances in its attempt to avoid the anthropomorphic tangles that such a study threatens to involve. It should construct a system that would meet the present multi-dimensions of its subsidiary sciences."[33]

For relevance regarding the practice of medicine, it's helpful to remember that from the scientific viewpoint, no matter the "first cause" of Creation, life-force is energy. The laws of physics and thermodynamics show that energy is conserved—it does not die, but merely changes form. Taken from this perspective, the idea that human life-force energy (or that of any living creature) can change form, once the physical body dies, is plausible. From a strictly scientific perspective, this continuation of life energy does not require a theological mediator or savior.

From the Hermetic perspective, whatever governs the subtle realms and higher octaves of space also governs the lower physical octaves of life.

What is helpful, if not required, is having a language that provides a road map for understanding the human being's connection to the cosmos. This is the relevance astrology brings to the process of responding to the larger cycles and hierarchical influence. It also facilitates understanding in the application of the doctrine of signatures to each human's life and, as applied by both Paracelsus and Agrippa Von Nettesheim (aka Henry Cornelius Agrippa), provides alchemical information regarding the process of healing.

Despite its controversy, we have to consider the longevity that has been demonstrated by astrology. While its popularity has waxed and waned over the centuries, like the moon, it remains ever present, orbiting the mainstream.[34] For this reason alone it deserves consideration as part of the historical, medical, and philosophical milieu of human inquiry.

TUNING IN FACILITATES TUNING UP

Whether we employ astrology or not, and despite the method we choose to engage in the healing process, for all of us there remains the opportunity to become better listeners to nature "out there" and to our own nature "in here" to support a more harmonious life. This attunement to nature is part of what allowed the ancient Chinese masters to develop their medicine. In his book *Music and Sound in the Healing Arts* (1987), John Beaulieu also emphasizes the importance of listening—to nature—and all that is around us. Specifically, he calls this "element listening," which he defines as the process of tuning into the music that arises in different environments out of the elements, a concept that is equally applicable to individuals.

He explains that when we envision a certain place in the mind's eye, we will also be thinking of its climate. For instance, Alaska is cold and windy, the Sahara desert hot and dry, and the Amazon hot, humid, and wet. Different geographic centers have their own "music" arising from the natural elements predominating in each region. The art of listening, however, comes about by trusting what arises out of the silence.

Music also creates environments. Element listening is looking through the reality around . . . music to the elements that give rise to that reality . . . In the past, the "gut-level" feelings of music were associated with human behavior and the qualities of natural elements . . . given the labels Ether (silence), Air, Fire, Water, and Earth . . . it is easy to be out of touch with the validity of our basic feeling responses . . . Listening on an elemental level requires a trust in our own primitive perceptions . . . All sounds rise from and lead back to silence . . . Silence is the key to the many adventures the world of sound has to offer . . . Through silence we are truly safe and free. We know the beginning and we know the end.[35]

Not only sound, but the silence to which it leads, is the key to reconciling all perceived dissonance, illness, darkness, chaos, and the like back to the self. Whether information shows up in chaos, silence, or harmony, its composer is the Infinite, and part of the greater process unfolding. When we remain unconscious to this process, we lose faith and invite fear, anger, and hatred in ourselves and in the world.

When we understand the construct by which all living beings connect—that feedback loop—and the means by which the Infinite communicates with us, we can participate with greater courage and receive ever-present renewal. This is what the language of cosmos (astrology) has to offer us.

ASTROLOGY REVEALS
HARMONIC RELATIONSHIPS

It bears repeating that healing is about relationships, and relationships require change and constant adjustment. More importantly, it must be remembered that the adjustments required in the process of healing stem from reciprocity among all living beings. In the cosmos, this is about harmonic relations among planets in our solar system; in the body, it is the harmonic relations among the organs and their energy pathways via the chakras and/or meridians. On the Earth, harmonic relations among all living creatures and the elements of the seasons keep things in balance.

Understanding the reciprocity from the minute and finite to the vast and infinite is essential for one who wishes to facilitate authentic medicine.

There are many valid systems of healing from which all of us may choose, and the reader is encouraged to seek further study in any area with which personal resonance is found. Likewise, it is important to realize that the example provided here is a mere shadow of the profound wisdom that accompanies the study and practice of any method if it is to be truly transformative and healing. I offer now the method I use because it synthesizes "my parts" (music, astrology, Chinese medicine) within the whole. Acutonics provides the framework whereby Earth and cosmic energies infuse the body with planetary music by way of the acupuncture mapping system.

FROM GALAXIES TO CELLS

Acutonics is an energy-based methodology that applies tuning forks to acupuncture points, trigger points, and points of pain to access the body's meridian and chakra energy systems. The tuning forks represent a natural harmonic series that is based on the orbital properties of the earth, moon, sun, and planets. While serving as clinical dean at the Northwest Institute of Acupuncture and Oriental Medicine (NIAOM) from 1995 to 2000, Donna Carey, a licensed acupuncturist, initially developed this approach. Carey was seeking a noninvasive therapy for acupuncturists to use with critically ill and needle-phobic patients. Research and practical application guided Carey to work with the cycles of nature as represented through the energy and quality of the planets, which she determined to be in alignment with Oriental medicine.[36]

With the assistance of Marjorie de Muynck (1953–2011), a shiatsu teacher and musician, and Paul and Jude Ponton, clinical faculty who were also at NIAOM at that time, this methodology was taught to students and introduced into fourteen community clinics. Since 1995 the Acutonics approach to integrative medicine has evolved into a full certification program through the efforts of Carey, Dr. Ellen F. Franklin, and Acutonics instructors worldwide, offering valuable new insights and research into this highly integrative care model.[37]

In its initial stages, the tuning forks used in Acutonics were based on Kepler's mathematical calculations of the orbital velocities of the planets, which were converted to Hertz (musical frequency) by Swiss mathematician Hans Cousto. Cousto's transposed frequencies were then incorporated into Acutonics early research with tuning forks. Carey went on to calculate additional frequencies for new planetary bodies based on dynamic rather than static models, which now encompasses a growing body of research supporting the efficacy of these frequencies in health care settings.[38]

What is particularly relevant about this body of work is that it provides a modern approach to integrative medicine that draws on ancient wisdom traditions: Taoism, Oriental medicine, music theory, depth psychology, archetypes, and modern science. The Acutonics methodology provides practitioners and clients with the ability to experience firsthand the living wisdom stemming from those themes I have explored throughout this book: the universe is musical, undivided, and transforming in orderly cycles.

> Although the strings of the universe are not being played by planetary gods, our ancestors' intuitions about the relationship of humanity to the vast universe that surrounded them was correct: that humanity is a microcosm, reflecting the macrocosm of the heavens—as above, so below; as without, so within. The key for advancement and evolution is to keep an open mind and heart, an open matrix that receives and honors the vast mystery and keen minds tuned into it through science and the arts, to participate and to fully understand that in the great cosmic symphony, we are all composers.[39]

ASTRO-HARMONIC MEDICINE

Analogous to the unique snowflake geometries, whose specific configuration is determined by the journey it makes through "cloudland," each person has a similar cosmic imprint unique to him or her. As the language that reveals an individual's signature, astrology is an apt tool for identifying where personal transformation may be needed most.

West describes the zodiac and sign combinations as being based upon duality, triplicity, and quadruplicity—echoing the polarities, modes, and elements per se.[40] He also states that the physical universe expresses itself in four principles: unity, polarity, relationship, and substantiality, noting that the "full actualization of all possibilities requires the working out of all combinations of Two, Three, and Four. This is accomplished in the twelve signs of the zodiac."[41]

Reminiscent of the alchemical response when different elements are mixed, the planetary vibrations combine to create an elixir of harmony. When seen from the perspective of cosmic order, the individual discovers that his/her own life, chaos notwithstanding, can still provide a road map back to wholeness and health.

In figure 9.4, a fictitious natal chart is shown as an example so that one can see the geometry (circles, triangles, squares in the center) of frozen harmonic relationships between the planetary archetypes. It will be readily apparent that there is great complexity here, and one can easily get lost in the archetypal, geometric maze.

At this point, it is helpful to review a few things from chapter 1. The natural chart is different from the natal chart. The former represents a geodesic picture with the four seasons on the angles, starting with the spring equinox, while the latter is based on the individual's birth time and place. Angles and planetary degrees (0–30 within each constellation) of the natal chart will vary within the twenty-four-hour cycle according to the constellation that emerges on the eastern horizon from earth's perspective. (Please refer to table 1.4 for a listing of the planetary and zodiac sign symbols. The chart shown here reveals many more than the original twelve archetypes, which may be examined in future publications.)

To bring this astrological maze "down to earth," metaphors are quite useful, as is the anthropomorphic metaphor so prevalent in ancient texts.

ANTHROPOMORPHIC PSYCHOLOGY: WHO, WHAT, AND WHERE

The planets represent our psychological function, analogous to "actors on a stage." The signs (constellations) in which they fall are analogous

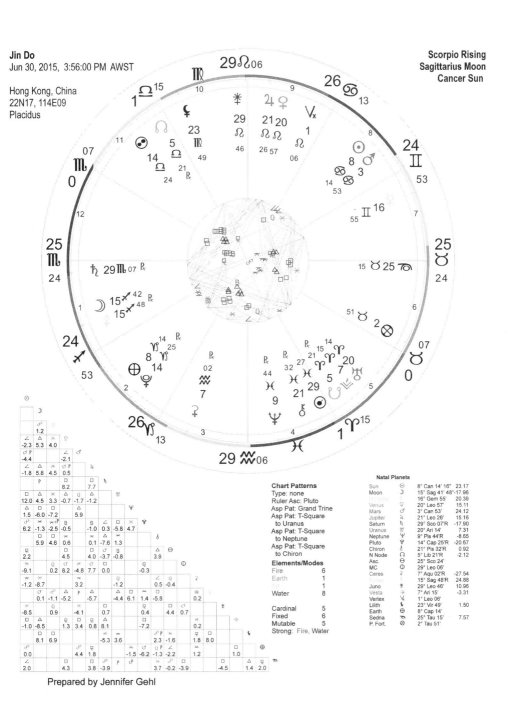

Fig. 9.4. Example of a fictitious natal chart.

to the role the actor is playing—what costume are they wearing? The houses represent the scenes of the play, with the chart in its entirety analogous to one's life. As the cycles continue, and planetary bodies move in the solar system, they trigger different areas of the natal signature. When this occurs, the interaction acts like a cosmic wake-up call, bringing forth different energies, and "raising up the humors" as it were (although, sometimes it doesn't feel too humorous to us!). What it does mean is that the "grand design" and cosmic order is inviting us to consciously participate in one's own journey toward health, for something requires conscious change and renewal.

Each person has the freedom to choose either to enhance the drama (ham it up by getting caught up in drama) or seek a more subtle way of working with these energies. It is entirely up to the individual, even if influenced by the reaction/response inherent in the elemental predominance.

The practice of "astro-harmonic" medicine is the process of interpreting which of these actors is "hamming it up" and "overacting" on other players. Bringing the psychological components together through music is one way to invite each to the proverbial conference table where their differences and dissonances may be heard, reconciled, and harmonized. This is a method analogous to harmonic homeopathy. As a marriage counselor might do for an argumentative couple, so too does the astro-harmonic healer facilitate mediation between the archetypes, thereby encouraging harmonic reciprocity. However, sometimes another arbiter needs to be incorporated to reverse a severe imbalance, either excess or deficiency.

How this affects one's health has to do with the physical and energetic functions these planets and archetypal relationships have for the individual. While there are "textbook" versions of how this can be achieved, the assessment is highly intuitive, individualized, and customizable. The other metaphor I like to use to describe one's natal chart is that of the individual's "key signature."

MUSICAL METAPHOR

When we consider that the word *person* traces back to the Greek roots *per* (meaning "through") and *son* (meaning "sound"), we realize that just as we are made of star stuff, we are also made of music. As the motion of the celestial bodies and their musical tones, continue to move through time, they create further harmonic relationships with the personal "key signature." Just as we have harmonic overtones in music, the transits create similar reverberations within, and in the life of, a person.

As a tool for maintaining harmony, sound can facilitate greater awareness of the feedback loops in the body and between humans and their environment. With practice, we can become more aware of subtle energy and, as that happens, gain greater appreciation of the essential roles dissonance and tension play in the healing process. Instead of dreading these feelings, we can use them to achieve lasting healing.

Recall the alchemical process that changes lead into gold, and the rebirth of self into a higher state of awareness. Recall, too, that those creations divisible by the golden ratio find infinite expression at the same time they are reconciled to the whole. We always have the choice to consciously work with, or deny and try to annihilate, that which brings challenge to our lives through its seeming lack of order. By recognizing the universal truth inherent in each living thing, including ourselves, we can develop greater awareness of mystery, the language of which is subtle energy.

What seems to "lurk in the shadows" holds potency beyond anything we might imagine because its source is the Infinite. Darkness (yin) represents the mystery, and is an ever present aspect of the undifferentiated wholeness. Not only is it a valid part of the conscious evolutionary process, it is a necessary aspect of the triune body's ability to absorb light, and evolve with it.

We have a golden opportunity, perhaps even an obligation, to remember all aspects of who we are, however mysterious and magical, and to let go of preconceived notions that keep us trapped in fearful responses. Darkness gives birth to light just as surely as night turns into day, and the path that leads you forward is the same that calls you back to yourself.

> *We shall not cease from exploration*
> *And the end of all our exploring*
> *Will be to arrive where we started*
> *And know the place for the first time.*
>   T. S. ELIOT, "LITTLE GIDDING"

AFTERWORD

Attune with the Moon
And Follow the Sun
Let trust be your guide
When each day is done

The chaos unfolding
Finds Order in Time
For Time follows Cycles
Of Heaven's Design

Push not the River
Seek Not to Divide
For All Things Are One
In One All Abide

JENNIFER GEHL

NOTES

CHAPTER 1.
ANCIENT COSMOLOGY

1. Dietrich, *The Culture of Astronomy*, 4.
2. Marino, *Christopher Columbus, The Last Templar*, 67, cited in Farrell, *Thrice Great Hermetica*, 142–143.
3. Farrell, *Thrice Great Hermetica*, 140–141.
4. Marino, *Christopher Columbus, The Last Templar*, 190, cited in Farrell, *Thrice Great Hermetica*, 144.
5. Ibid., 192, in Farell, *Thrice Great Hermetica*, 144.
6. Farrell, *Thrice Great Hermetica*, 146.
7. Hammer, "What is Beneath the Temple Mount?"
8. Hall, *Secret Teachings*, 579.
9. Ibid.
10. Ibid., 582.
11. Ibid., 581–582.
12. Dietrich, *The Culture of Astronomy*, 5.
13. Ibid., 364–367.
14. Dietrich, *The Origin of Culture*, 63.
15. Ibid., 63–64.
16. Pinkham, *Return of Serpents*, 161.
17. Ibid.
18. Dietrich, *The Culture of Astronomy*, 142.
19. Ibid, 439.
20. Blavatsky, *Isis Unveiled*, 398.

21. Pinkham, *Return of Serpents,* 233.

22. *New-York Tribune* cited in Blavatsky, *Isis Unveiled* (1877).

23. Ibid.

24. Ibid., 19.

25. Blavatsky, *Isis Unveiled: Secrets,* 243.

26. Dietrich, *Culture of Astronomy,* 90.

27. Ibid., 115.

28. Ibid., 114.

29. Ibid.

30. Dietrich, *The Origin of Culture,* 200.

31. Dietrich, *Culture of Astronomy,* 115.

32. Ibid., 118.

33. Ibid., 117.

34. Ibid.

35. Ibid., 118.

36. Churchward, *Lost Continent,* 27.

37. Blavatsky, *The Secret Doctrine,* 12, 20.

38. Narby, *Cosmic Serpent,* 83.

39. Pinkham, *Return of Serpents,* 232.

40. Ibid., 270–271.

41. Farrell, *Philosopher's Stone,* 33–34.

42. Farebrother, *Astrology Decoded,* 9.

43. Kirk, *Influence of Zodiac,* 19.

44. Ibid., 26–27.

45. Agrippa, *Agrippa's Occult Philosophy,* 119.

46. Boehme, *The Signature of All Things,* 100–105.

47. Agrippa, *Agrippa's Occult Philosophy,* 110–111.

48. Ibid., 119–120.

49. Ibid., 109.

50. Ibid., 107–109.

CHAPTER 2.
HISTORY OF HERMETIC MEDICINE

1. Lumpkin, *The Books of Enoch,* 186.

2. Blavatsky, *The Secret Doctrine,* 220.

3. Freke and Gandy, *The Hermetica,* 7.

4. NIH, "Greek Medicine."

5. Ferguson, *Music of Pythagoras,* 52.

6. Hall, *Secret Teachings,* 15.

7. Ibid., 199.

8. Ibid., 505.

9. Ibid., 197.

10. Ibid., 251.

11. NIH, "Greek Medicine."

12. Nutton, *Ancient Medicine,* 116.

13. Ibid., 116–117.

14. Internet Encyclopedia of Philosophy, "Galen."

15. Ibid.

16. Ibid.

17. Abu-Asab, Amri, and Micozzi, *Avicenna's Medicine,* 5.

18. Paracelsus, *Hermetic and Alchemical Writings,* 29.

19. Ibid.

20. Abu-Asab, Mones, Amri, and Micozzi, *Avicenna's Medicine.*

21. Ibid.

22. Ibid., 135.

23. Strehlow and Hertzka, *Bingen's Medicine,* xxvi.

24. Ibid., x.

25. Ibid., xx.

26. Ibid.

27. Hall, *Secret Teachings,* 484.

28. Ibid., 485.

29. Hall, *Paracelsus: His Mystical and Medical Philosophy,* 15.

30. Hall, *Secret Teachings,* 332.

31. Ibid, 344.

32. Culpeper, *Astrological Judgement of Diseases,* 31.

33. Micozzi and Gehl, "Nutrition, Hydration, and Diet Therapies," in Micozzi, *Fundamentals.*

34. Ergil, "Tibetan Medicine," in Micozzi, *Fundamentals.*

CHAPTER 3.
COSMOLOGICAL ROOTS OF YIN AND YANG

1. Acharya, *The Christ Conspiracy,* 105.

2. Marrs, *Our Occulted History,* in Hardy, *DNA of Gods,* 10–11.

3. Hardy, *DNA of Gods,* 11.

4. Micozzi, *Celestial Healing,* 14.

5. Lewis, *Flood Myths,* 120.

6. Scranton, *China's Cosmological Prehistory,* 41.

7. Lewis, *Flood Myths,* 112.

8. Micozzi, *Celestial Healing,* 19.

9. Wilhelm and Baynes, *The I Ching, or Book of Changes,* 328.

10. Wong, *Tales of the Dancing Dragon,* 14–15.

11. Scranton, *China's Cosmological Prehistory,* 42.

12. Jackson, *Christianity before Christ,* 10.

13. Scranton, *China's Cosmological Prehistory,* 40.

14. Veggi and Davidson, *Book of Doors,* 76.

15. Ibid., 76.

16. Jackson, *Christianity before Christ,* 10.

17. Hardy, *DNA of Gods,* 22.

18. Ibid., 3.

19. Ibid., 4.

20. Ibid., 5.

21. Ibid., 5, 108.

22. Ibid., 108.

23. Ibid.

24. Ibid., 106.

25. Ibid., 203.

26. Ibid., 204.

27. Ibid., 210.

28. Hardy, *DNA of Gods,* 98.

29. Hardy, *DNA of Gods,* 47.

30. Ibid.

31. Tellinger, *African Temples,* 3, 54, 128.

32. Pinkham, *Return of Serpents,* 188–190.

33. Wilhelm and Baynes, *The I Ching, or Book of Changes.*

34. Scranton, *Cosmological Origins of Myth,* 150.

35. Ibid., 151.

36. Ibid., 155.

37. Ibid., 153.

38. Ibid., 154.

39. Ibid.
40. Ibid., 153.
41. Lewis, *Flood Myths,* 111.
42. Veggi and Davidson, *Book of Doors,* 176.
43. Ibid., 9.
44. Ibid., 14–15.
45. Man Ho and O'Brien, *Eight Immortals.*
46. Ibid., 9.
47. Ibid., 11.
48. Ibid., 14.
49. Campbell, *Oriental Mythology,* 438–439.
50. Pinkham, *Return of Serpents,* 138.
51. Ibid.
52. Ibid., 138.
53. Ibid., 139.
54. Ibid., 140.
55. Ibid., 140–141.
56. Ibid., 140.
57. Micozzi, *Celestial Healing,* 16.
58. Mitchell, *Tao Te Ching,* 48.
59. Wong, *Tales of the Dancing Dragon,* 11–13.
60. Jaeger, "A Geomedical Approach to Chinese Medicine," 30.
61. Dietrich, *The Culture of Astronomy,* 389.
62. Jaeger, "A Geomedical Approach to Chinese Medicine," 32.
63. Ellis and Wiseman, *Grasping the Wind,* 425–427.
64. Maciocia, *Foundations of Chinese Medicine,* 21.
65. Ibid., 279.
66. Wong, *Tales of the Dancing Dragon,* 17.
67. Ibid., 19.

CHAPTER 4.
THE FOUR BUILDING BLOCKS OF THE COSMOS

1. Dietrich, *The Culture of Astronomy,* 227.
2. Lewis, *Flood Myths,* 111.
3. Veggi and Davidson, *Book of Doors,* 44.
4. Red Star and Goodluck, *Star Ancestors,* 6.

5. Ibid., 29.

6. Ibid., 65.

7. Ibid., 69.

8. Blavatsky, *The Secret Doctrine,* 199.

9. Ibid., 200.

10. Wasserman, *Art and Symbols of the Occult,* in Dietrich, *The Culture of Astronomy,* 227.

11. Agrippa, *Natural Magic,* 274.

12. Blavatsky, *The Secret Doctrine* (1917), 125.

13. Heath, *Sacred Number,* 89.

14. Levi, *Dogma and Ritual,* 49–50.

15. Ibid., 46–47.

16. Blavatsky, *The Secret Doctrine* (2009), 226–227.

17. Massey, *Historical Jesus,* 114–116.

18. Levi, *Dogma and Ritual,* 45.

19. Krakowski, "How the Hexagrams."

20. Levi in Blavatsky, *Isis Unveiled* (1877), 87.

21. Krakowski, "How the Hexagrams."

22. Shah, *Astrology Realized,* loc. 3032 (e-book).

CHAPTER 5. THE HEXAGON PHENOMENON

1. Blanchard, *The Snowflake Man,* 22.

2. Ibid.

3. Suddath, "Vibration, Energy, and Water," 1–3.

4. Linus Pauling Institute, "Linus Pauling Biography."

5. Nobel Prize Media, "Linus Pauling—Biographical."

6. Nakada, "Neuroscience of Water Molecules."

7. Kepler, *The Six-Cornered Snowflake,* 33.

8. Snow Crystals, "Snowflake Branching."

9. Blanchard, *The Snowflake Man,* 153.

10. Haramein, Facebook status posted December 5, 2013.

11. Schneider, *Beginner's Guide,* 193.

12. Ibid. 189–196.

13. Haramein, Facebook status posted December 5, 2013.

14. Cosmometry, "Vector Equilibrium."

15. "Fractal Holographic Universe."

16. Ibid.

17. Ibid.

18. Ibid.

19. Schneider, *Beginner's Guide,* 201.

20. "Fractal Holographic Universe."

21. The Resonance Project, Module 4, "Unified Field."

22. Ibid.

23. hiup.org/publications.

24. The Resonance Project, n.d.

25. Boerst, *J. Johannes Kepler,* 37.

26. Ibid., 38.

27. Ibid., 41.

28. Ibid., 70.

29. Kepler, *Harmony of the World,* 6.

30. Boerst, *J. Johannes Kepler,* 105.

31. Ibid, 43.

32. Today In Science, "Johannes Kepler's Quotations."

33. Wilhelm, *The Secret of the Golden Flower,* 8.

34. Ibid.

35. Ibid., 11, 65.

36. Haramein, Facebook status posted December 5, 2013.

37. Krakowski, "How the Hexagrams."

38. Ibid.

39. SciTechDaily, "Atomic Bond Types."

40. Hall, *Secret Teachings.*

CHAPTER 6.
COSMIC LIGHT IN INNER AND OUTER SPACE

1. *The Secrets of Astrology.*

2. Bynum, *Dark Light Consciousness,* 23.

3. Ibid., 28.

4. Ibid.

5. Ibid.

6. Ibid., 29.

7. French, *Hidden Geometry,* 107.

8. Bynum, *Dark Light Consciousness,* 118–119.

9. Ibid., 30.

10. Hall, *Melchizedek and the Mystery of Fire,* 55.

11. Bynum, *Dark Light Consciousness,* 84.

12. Ibid., 81–82.

13. Ibid., 82.

14. Schwaller de Lubicz, *Temple in Man,* 17.

15. Anderson, *Astrology of Old Testament,* 16–18.

16. Ibid., 50.

17. Ibid., 285.

18. Ibid., 36.

19. Ibid., 180.

20. *Essai sur la Philosophie des Sciences* vol. 2, 103–104 in Schwaller de Lubicz, *Temple in Man,* 19.

21. See Livio's *The Golden Ratio,* 21, for alternative explanation of 666.

22. Anderson, *Astrology of Old Testament,* 36–37.

23. Ibid., 20.

24. West, *Serpent in the Sky,* 1.

25. http://www.etymonline.com/index.php?

26. Hall, *Melchizedek.*

27. Ibid., 13.

28. Wilcock, *Hidden Science,* 301–302.

29. Hall, *Melchizedek,* 14–15.

30. Levi, *History of Magic,* in Hall, *Melchizedek,* 15–16.

31. Marrs, *Our Occulted History,* in Hardy, *DNA of the Gods,* 10–11.

32. West, *The Serpent in the Sky,* 2.

33. Anderson, *Astrology of Old Testament,* 8–9.

34. Joseph, *Before Atlantis,* 143.

35. Hall, *Occult Anatomy of Man,* 6.

36. Ibid, 12–13.

37. Seawright, "Egypt: Amentet, Goddess of the Dead."

38. Schwaller de Lubicz, *Sacred Science,* 145–148.

39. Ibid., 148.

40. Schwaller de Lubicz, *Temple in Man,* 48.

41. Hall, *Occult Anatomy,* 18.

42. Bynum, *Dark Light Consciousness,* 98–99.

43. Ibid., 232.

44. Vaid, *Brahmandic Gyanum: Universal Knowledge,* 32.

45. Hall, *Melchizedek,* 32.

46. Anderson, *Astrology of the Old Testament,* 181.

47. Clogstoun-Willmott, *Western Astrology and Chinese Medicine,* 59.

48. Hall, *Occult Anatomy,* 24, 33.

49. Ibid, 21.

50. Ibid, 19.

51. Wilcock, *Hidden Science,* 18.

52. Bailey, *Esoteric Healing,* 19.

53. Willner, *Perfect Horoscope,* 239–247.

54. Micozzi, *Fundamentals of Complementary and Alternative Medicine,* 335.

CHAPTER 7.
PHI-LOSOPHY: THE MEAN BETWEEN
THE EXTREMES

1. Olsen, *Golden Section,* 6.

2. Ibid., 55.

3. James, *Music of Spheres, 36.*

4. Nature's Word, *Introduction to Phi.*

5 Ibid.

6. Ibid.

7. Ibid.

8. Livio, *Golden Ratio,* 35.

9. Ibid., 36.

10. Guthrie, *Pythagorean Sourcebook and Library,* 19.

11. Ibid., 19-20.

12. Ibid., 21.

13. Ibid., 35.

14. Ibid., 34.

15. Ibid., 28.

16. Ibid., 29.

17. Teia, "Ancient Babylonian Use."

18. Guthrie, *Pythagorean Sourcebook and Library,* 25.

19. Ibid.

20. Ibid., 29.

21. Ibid., 25.

22. Ibid.

23. Theon of Smyrna, *Mathematics Useful for Understanding Plato,* in Guthrie, *Pythagorean Sourcebook and Library,* 318.

24. Ibid.

25. Guthrie, *Pythagorean Sourcebook and Library,* 21.

26. Ibid.

27. James, *Music of the Spheres,* 38.

28. Guthrie, *Pythagorean Sourcebook and Library,* 25.

29. Hall, *Secret Teachings,* 252.

30. Ibid.

31. *Life of Pythagoras,* in Livio, *The Golden Ratio,* 29.

32. Hall, *Secret Teachings,* 203.

33. Ibid.

34. Ibid., 203–205.

35. Olsen, *Golden Section,* 46.

36. Ferguson, *Music of Pythagoras,* 133–134.

37. Ibid., 135.

38. Ibid., 139.

39. Ibid.

40. James, *Music of Spheres,* 35.

41. Ibid.

42. Olsen, *Golden Section,* 54.

43. James, *Music of Spheres,* 131.

44. Olsen, *Golden Section,* 55.

45. Ibid., 54.

46. Ibid.

47. Ibid.

48. Ferguson, *Music of Pythagoras,* 133.

49. Olsen, *Golden Section,* 55.

CHAPTER 8.
NATURE'S SPIN: A SOUND EFFECT?

1. Tompkins and Bird, *Secret Life of Plants,* 162.

2 Jenny, *Cymatics,* 21.

3. Ibid., 34.

4. Ibid., 27–29.

5. Ibid., 28.

6. Ibid.

7. Ibid., 28, 210.

8. Ibid., 63–64.

9. Ibid., 181.

10. Ibid.

11. Ibid., 214.

12. Berendt, *World is Sound*, 76.

13. Capra and Luisi, *Systems View of Life*, 170.

14. Ibid., 163.

15. Watson and Lovelock, *Biological Homeostasis*, in Capra and Luisi, *Systems View of Life*, 165.

16. Capra and Luisi, *Systems View of Life*, 91.

17. Ibid., 172.

18. Ibid., 178.

19. Hemenway, *Divine Proportion*, 127.

20. Ibid.

21. Capra and Luisi, *Systems View of Life*, 176.

22. Posamentier and Lehmann, *Glorious Golden Ratio*, 255.

23. Ibid.

24. Ibid.

25. Ibid., 263.

26. Ibid.

27. Ibid., 265.

28. Ibid.

29. Ibid.

30. Capra and Luisi, *Systems View of Life*, 169.

31. Stewart, *The Mathematics of Life*, in Capra and Luisi, *Systems View of Life*, 177.

32. Tompkins and Bird, *Secret Life of Plants*, 161.

33. Ibid.

34. Ibid.

35. Ibid., 161–162.

36. Jenny, *Cymatics*.

37. Ibid., 255–256.

38. Scott, "Birds, Thermals, and Soaring Flight."

39. Livio, *Golden Ratio*, 120.

40. Ibid.

41. Scott, "Birds, Thermals, and Soaring Flight."

42. French, *Hidden Geometry,* 46.

43. Olsen, *Golden Section,* 46.

44. Ibid.

45. Ibid.

CHAPTER 9.
THE FUTURE AWAITS OUR RETURN

1. Schwaller de Lubicz, *Sacred Science,* 184–185.

2. Ibid.

3. Schneider, *Beginner's Guide,* 125.

4. Ibid.

5. Ibid.

6. Capra, *Learning from Leonardo,* 129.

7. Ibid., 136.

8. Ibid., 140.

9. Ibid.

10. Ibid., 139.

11. Ibid., 145.

12. Ibid., 219.

13. Laurenza, "La grammatica delle forme," in Capra, *Learning from Leonardo,* 142.

14. Capra, *Learning from Leonardo,* 147.

15. Ibid., 151.

16. Ibid., 175.

17. Ibid.

18. Bynum, *Dark Light Consciousness,* 30.

19. Capra, *Learning from Leonardo,* 281.

20. Ibid., 284.

21. Freke and Gandy, *Hermetica,* 48.

22. Ibid., 30–32.

23. Schneider, *Beginner's Guide,* 127–128.

24. Freke and Gandy, *Hermetica,* 87.

25. Scranton, *China's Cosmological Prehistory,* 7.

26. Ibid.

27. Hurtak, *The Book of Knowledge,* 523.

28. Ibid.

29. Freke and Gandy, *Hermetica,* 51–52.

30. Boehme, *The Signature of All Things,* 12.

31. Buchanan, *Doctrine of Signatures,* 32–33.

32. Ibid., 143.

33. Ibid., 145.

34. Farebrother, *Astrology Decoded,* 9.

35. Beaulieu, *Music and Sound,* 16–17.

36. Carey, et.al, *Acutonics From Galaxies*; and Franklin, "Acutonics Self Care Program."

37. Franklin, "Acutonics Self Care Program"; Carey, et.al, *Acutonics From Galaxies*; and Carey and de Muynck, *There's No Place.*

38. Carey et al., *Acutonics From Galaxies,* 88–89.

39. Ibid., 47.

40. West, *Serpent in the Sky,* 53.

41. Ibid.

BIBLIOGRAPHY

Abu-Asab, Mones, Hakima Amri, and Marc S. Micozzi. *Avicenna's Medicine: A New Translation of the 11th-Century Canon with Practical Applications for Integrative Health Care.* Rochester, Vt.: Inner Traditions International, 2013.

Acharya, S. *The Christ Conspiracy: The Greatest Story Ever Sold.* Kempton, Ill.: Adventures Unlimited Press, 1999.

Agrippa, Cornelius. *Agrippa's Occult Philosophy: Natural Magic.* Edited by Willis F. Whitehead. Mineola, N.Y.: Dover Publications, Inc., 2006.

Ampère, André-Marie. *Essai sur la Philosophie des Sciences (Essai sur la Philosophie des Sciences).* Paris: Bacheler, Imprimeur-Libraire pour les Sciences, 1834.

Anderson, Karl. *Astrology of the Old Testament or the Lost World Regained.* Whitefish, Mont.: Kessinger Publishing, 1892.

Bailey, Alice A. *Esoteric Healing: A Treatise on the Seven Rays, Volume IV.* Lucis Trust, 1953, 1981. http://researchnfeh.org/wp-content/uploads/2015/04/Esoteric-Healing-a-Treatise-on-the-Seven-Rays-Vol-4.pdf.

Beaulieu, John. *Music and Sound in the Healing Arts.* Barrytown, N.Y.: Station Hill Press, Inc., 1987.

Berendt, Joachim-Ernst. *The World is Sound: Nada Brahma: Music and the Landscape of Consciousness.* Rochester, Vt.: Destiny Books, 1983.

Bibliotecapleyades. "The Pagan Origins of Jesus Christ and Christianity." www.bibliotecapleyades.net/biblianazar/esp_biblianazar_33.htm. Accessed January 15, 2015.

Blanchard, Duncan C. *The Snowflake Man: A Biography of Wilson A. Bentley.* Blacksburg, Va: McDonald & Woodward Publishing Co., 1998.

————. "Johannes Kepler's Six-Cornered Snowflakes." *Jericho Historical Society* 17 (2011). http://snowflakebentley.com/WBnews.htm#n17. Accessed February 1, 2015.

Blavatsky, H. P. *Isis Unveiled: A Master Key to the Mysteries of Ancient and Modern Science and Theology.* New York: Cambridge University Press, 1877. Digitally printed version 2012.

————. *Isis Unveiled: A Master Key to the Mysteries of Ancient and Modern Science and Theology.* Vol. 1. 6th ed. New York: J.W. Bouton, 1892.

————. *Isis Unveiled: Secrets of the Ancient Wisdom Tradition, Madame Blavatsky's First Work.* Abridged and annotated by Michael Gomes. Wheaton, Illinois: The Theosophical Publishing House, 1972, 1997.

————. *The Secret Doctrine.* Abridged and annotated by Michael Gomes. New York: Jeremy B. Tarcher/Penguin, 2009.

————. *The Secret Doctrine: The Synthesis of Science, Religion, and Philosophy.* Vol. 2. Point Loma, Calif.: The Aryan Theosophical Press, 1917.

Boerst, William. *J. Johannes Kepler: Discovering the Laws of Celestial Motion.* Greensboro, N.C.: Morgan Reynolds Publishing, Inc., 2003.

Boehme, Jacob. *The Signature of All Things.* 2nd ed. London: Forgotten Books, 2008.

Bohm, David, and F. David Peat. *Science, Order, and Creativity.* New York: Bantam Books, 1987.

Buchanan, Scott. *The Doctrine of Signatures: A Defense of Theory in Medicine.* 2nd ed. Introduction by Peter P. Mayock, Jr. Chicago: University of Illinois Press, 1991.

Bynum, Edward B. *Dark Light Consciousness: Melanin, Serpent Power, and the Luminous Matrix of Reality.* Rochester, Vt.: Inner Traditions, 2012.

Campbell, Joseph. *Oriental Mythology (The Masks of God).* New York: Penguin Books, 1976.

Capra, Fritjof. *Learning from Leonardo: Decoding the Notebooks of a Genius.* San Francisco: Berrett-Koehler Publishers, 2013.

Capra, Fritjof, and Pier Luigi Luisi. *The Systems View of Life: A Unifying Vision.* Cambridge, UK: Cambridge University Press, 2014.

Carey, Donna, and Marjorie de Muynck. *There's No Place Like Ohm.* Vadito, N.Mex: Devachan Press, Inc, 2007.

Carey, Donna, Ellen F. Franklin, Judith Ponton, Paul Ponton, and MichelAngelo. *Acutonics From Galaxies to Cells: Planetary Science, Harmony, and Medicine.* Llano, N.Mex.: Devachan Press, 2010.

Churchward, James. *The Lost Continent of Mu.* New York: Paperback Library, Inc., 1968.

Clogstoun-Willmott, Jonathan. *Western Astrology and Chinese Medicine.* New York: Destiny Books, 1985.

Cosmometry. "Vector Equilibrium and Isotropic Vector Matrix." http://cosmometry.net/vector-equilibrium-&-isotropic-vector-matrix. Last modified 2014. Accessed February 1, 2015.

Cousto, Hans. *The Cosmic Octave: Origin of Harmony.* Mendocino, Calif.: LifeRhythm, 1988.

Culpeper, Nicholas. *Astrological Judgement of Diseases from the Decumbiture of the Sick.* Bel Air, Md.: The Astrology Center of America, 2003.

Dietrich, Thomas K. *The Culture of Astronomy.* Minneapolis, Minn.: Bascom Publishing, 2011.

———. *The Origin of Culture and Civilization.* Austin, Tex.: TurnKey Press, 2005.

Ellis, Andrew W., and Nigel Wiseman. *Grasping the Wind.* Brookline, Mass: Paradigm Publications, 1989.

Emoto, Masaru. *The Hidden Messages in Water.* Translated by David Thayne. Hillsboro, Ore.: Beyond Words Publishing, Inc., 2004.

———. "Dr. Masaru Emoto." http://www.masaru-emoto.net/english/emoto.htm. Accessed February 14, 2015.

Ergil, Kevin V. "Tibetan Medicine." In *Fundamentals of Complementary and Alternative Medicine,* 5th ed., by Marc S. Micozzi. St. Louis, Mo.: Elsevier Saunders, 2015.

Etymonline (Online Etymology Dictionary). "Pyre." http://www.etymonline.com/index.php?allowed_in_frame=0&search=pyre. Accessed July 21, 2016.

Evolution TV. *Secrets of the Universe.* (September 3, 2013). www.youtube.com/watch?v=B5fegQuv6s8

Farebrother, Sue M. *Astrology Decoded: A Step-by-Step Guide to Learning Astrology.* London: Rider/Ebury Publishing, 2013.

Farrell, Joseph P. *The Philosopher's Stone: Alchemy and the Secret Research for Exotic Matter.* Port Townsend, Wash.: Feral House, 2009.

———. *Thrice Great Hermetica and the Janus Age.* Kempton, Illinois: Adventures Unlimited Press, 2014.

Ferguson, Kitty. *The Music of Pythagoras.* New York: Walker and Company, 2008.

Fractal Holographic Universe. "The Fractal Holographic Universe." http://holofractal.net/the-holofractographic-universe/. Accessed February 5, 2015.

Franklin, Ellen F. "Acutonics Self-care Program and Stress: Multiple Case Study Exploration of an Intervention to Ameliorate Symptoms of Severe Stress and Compassion Fatigue in Nurses." Ph.D. diss., Saybrook University, 2014.

Freke, Timothy, and Peter Gandy. *The Hermetica: The Lost Wisdom of the Pharaohs.* New York: Penguin Group, Inc., 1997.

French, Karen L. *The Hidden Geometry of Life: The Science and Spirituality of Nature.* London: Watkins Publishing Ltd., 2012.

Gallagher, Christine M. "The Effects of Acutonics on Perceptions of Joy." Unpublished doctoral dissertation. Clayton College of Natural Health, 2010.

Good, Maren. "Pythagoras, the Music of the Spheres, and its Relevance in the 21st Century in Health, Healing and Conscious Evolution." Unpublished master's thesis. Graduate Institute, 2012.

Guthrie, Kenneth Sylvan, compiler and trans. *The Pythagorean Sourcebook and Library: An Anthology of Ancient Writings Which Relate to Pythagoras and Pythagorean Philosophy.* Grand Rapids, Mich.: Phanes Press, 1987.

Hall, Manly P. *Melchizedek and the Mystery of Fire.* Los Angeles: Philosophical Research Society, 1996.

———. *The Occult Anatomy of Man And Occult Masonry.* Los Angeles: Philosophical Research Society, 1997.

———. *Paracelsus: His Mystical and Medical Philosophy.* Los Angeles: Philosophical Research Society, 1997.

———. *The Secret Teachings of All Ages.* New York: Jeremy P. Tarcher/Penguin, 2003.

Hammer, Joshua. "What is Beneath the Temple Mount?" *Smithsonian Magazine,* 2011. http://www.smithsonianmag.com/history/what-is-beneath-the-temple-mount-920764. Accessed July 16, 2016.

Hardy, Chris H. *DNA of the Gods: The Anunnaki Creation of Eve and the Alien Battle for Humanity.* Rochester, Vt.: Bear and Company, 2014.

Haramein, Nassim. Facebook photo posted December 5, 2014. www.facebook.com/Nassim.Haramein.official/photos/a.112729698918297.1073741828.106168786241055/312489982275600.

Haramein, Nassim. Facebook status posted December 5, 2013. www.facebook.com/Nassim.Haramein.official/posts/192454530945813.

Heath, Richard. *Sacred Number and the Origins of Civilization: The Unfolding of History through the Mystery of Number.* Rochester, Vt.: Inner Traditions, 2007.

Hemenway, Priya. *Divine Proportion: ϕ PHI In Art, Nature, and Science.* New York: Sterling Publishing, 2005.

Hurtak, J. J. *The Book of Knowledge: The Keys of Enoch.* Ava, Miss.: The Academy for Future Science, 1977.

Hyper Physics. "Black Hole Conditions." http://hyperphysics.phy-astr.gsu.edu /hbase/astro/blkhol.htm. Accessed February 9, 2015.

Internet Encyclopedia of Philosophy. "Galen." www.iep.utm.edu/galen. Accessed February 22, 2015.

Jackson, John G. *Christianity Before Christ.* Austin, Tex.: American Atheist Press, 1985.

Jaeger, Stephen. "A Geomedical Approach to Chinese Medicine: The Origin of the Yin-Yang Symbol." *Intech: Science, Technology, and Medicine open access publisher* (2012). Accessed July 18, 2016. doi: 10-5772/27241.

James, Jamie. *The Music of the Spheres: Music, Science and the Natural Order of the Universe.* New York: Springer-Verlag, 1993.

Jenny, Hans. *Cymatics.* Newmarket, N.H.: MACROmedia Publishing, 2001.

Joseph, Frank. *Before Atlantis: 20 Million Years of Human and Pre-Human Cultures.* Rochester, Vt.: Bear & Company, 2013.

Kepler, Johannes. *The Six-Cornered Snowflake: A New Year's Gift.* Philadelphia: Paul Dry Books, Inc., 2010. Originally published in 1611.

———. *The Harmony of the World.* Translated by Charles Glenn Wallis, 2014.

Kirk, Eleanor. *The Influence of the Zodiac upon Human Life.* Albuquerque, N.Mex.: Sun Publishing Company, 1981.

Krakowski, Steven. "How the Hexagrams (Kua) Are Assigned to the Genetic Code Codons." Bibliotecapleyades. Last modified 1996. www .bibliotecapleyades.net/ciencia/occultgeneticcode/table04.html. Accessed February 2, 2015.

Laurenza, Domenico. "La grammatica delle forme." In *La mente di Leonardo,* edited by Paolo Galluzzi, 152–57. Exhibition catalogue. Florence, Italy: Giunti, 2006.

Levi, Eliphas. *The History of Magic: Its Procedure, Rites and Mysteries.* Translated by Arthur Edward Waite. Calgary, Canada: Theophania Publishing, 2012. First published 1913.

———. *The Dogma and Ritual of High Magic: Book One.* Translated by Arthur Edward Waite. San Diego, Calif.: St. Alban Press, 2011.

Lewis, Mark Edward. *The Flood Myths of Early China.* Albany, N.Y.: State University of New York Press, 2006.

Linus Pauling Institute. "Linus Pauling Biography." Oregon State University,

2015. http://lpi.oregonstate.edu/linus-pauling-biography. Accessed February 2, 2015.

Livio, Mario. *The Golden Ratio: The Story of Phi, The World's Most Astonishing Number.* New York: Broadway Books, 2002.

Lumpkin, Joseph. *The Books of Enoch: The Angels, The Watchers, and the Nephilim: (With Extensive Commentary on the Three Books of Enoch, the Fallen Angels, the Calendar of Enoch and Daniel's Prophecy).* 2nd ed. Blountsville, Alabama: Fifth Estate Publishers, Inc., 2011.

Maciocia, Giovanni. *The Foundations of Chinese Medicine: A Comprehensive Text for Acupuncturists and Herbalists.* London: Churchill Livingstone, 1989.

Man Ho, Kwok, and Joanne O'Brien. *The Eight Immortals of Taoism: Legends and Fables of Popular Taoism.* New York: Penguin Group, 1990.

Marino, Ruggero. *Christopher Columbus, The Last Templar.* Rochester, Vt.: Destiny Books, 2005.

Marrs, Jim. *Our Occulted History: Do the Global Elite Conceal Ancient Aliens?* New York: Harper Collins, 2013.

Martineau, John. *A Little Book of Coincidence in the Solar System.* New York: Bloomsbury USA, 2006.

Massey, Gerald. *The Historical Jesus and the Mythical Christ: Separating Fact from Fiction.* Escondido, Calif.: The Book Tree, 2000.

Micozzi, Marc S. *Celestial Healing.* London: Singing Dragon, 2011.

———. *Fundamentals of Complementary and Alternative Medicine.* 5th ed. St. Louis, Mo.: Elsevier Saunders, 2015.

Micozzi, Marc S., and Jennifer Gehl. "Nutrition, Hydration, and Diet Therapies." In *Fundamentals of Complementary and Alternative Medicine,* 5th ed., by Marc S. Micozzi. St. Louis, Mo.: Elsevier Saunders, 2015.

Mitchell, Stephen, translator. *Tao Te Ching: A New English Version.* By Lao Tzu. New York: Harper Perrenial, 1988.

Nakada, Tsutomu. "Neuroscience of Water Molecules: A Salute to Professor Linus Carl Pauling." *Springer-Cytotechnology* (2009). Accessed February 5, 2015. doi: 10.1007/s10616-009-9216-x.

Natures-word.com. n.d. *Introduction to Phi/The Golden Proportion.* Accessed July 22, 2016. www.natures-word.com/sacred-geometry/phi-the-golden -proportion/introduction-to-phi-the-golden-proportion.

Narby, James. *Cosmic Serpent: DNA and the Origins of Knowledge.* New York: Jeremy P. Tarcher/Putnam, 1998.

National Institute of Health (NIH). "Greek Medicine." www.nlm.hih.gov /hmd/greek/greek_oath.htm. Accessed December 12, 2014.

Nobel Prize Media AB. "Linus Pauling—Biographical." www.nobelprice.org /nobel_prizes/peace/laureates/1962/pauling-bio.htm. Accessed February 5, 2015.

Nutton, Vivian. *Ancient Medicine.* New York: Routledge, 2013.

Olsen, Scott. *The Golden Section: Nature's Greatest Secret.* New York: Bloomsbury USA, 2006.

Paracelsus. *The Hermetic and Alchemical Writings of Aureolus Philippus Theophrastus Bombast, of Hohenheim, Called Paracelsus The Great.* Translated and edited by Arthur Edward Waite. Mansfield, Conn.: Martino Publishing, 2009.

Pinkham, Mark Amaru. *The Return of the Serpents of Wisdom.* Kempton, Ill.: Adventures Unlimited Press, 1997.

Ponton, Judith, and Paul Ponton. *Acutonics from Galaxies to Cells: Case Study Companion Guide.* Vadito, N.Mex.: Devachan Press, 2010.

Life of Pythagoras by Porphyry. Translated by Kenneth S. Guthrie. Alpine, N.J.: Platonist Press, 1919.

Posamentier, Alfred S., and Ingmar Lehmann. *The Glorious Golden Ratio.* Amherst, N.Y.: Prometheus Books, 2012.

Red Star, Nancy, and Harriet Goodluck. "Weaving the Web is the Way of Women." In *Star Ancestors: Extraterrestrial Contact in the Native American Tradition.* Rochester, Vt.: Bear and Company, 2012.

Red Star, Nancy, and Mali Keating. "We Wander This World With a Purpose: Law of Light-Sound." In *Star Ancestors: Extraterrestrial Contact in the Native American Tradition.* Rochester, Vt.: Bear and Company, 2012.

Red Star, Nancy, and Troy Lang. "The Star Nations Are Here To Help Us: Healing the Four Races." In *Star Ancestors: Extraterrestrial Contact in the Native American Tradition.* Rochester, Vt.: Bear and Company, 2012.

The Resonance Project. "Module 4: The Holographic Network of Spacetime." http://academy.resonance.is/topic/4-5-1-the-holographic-network-of-space-time. Accessed July 15, 2015.

———. "Module 4: Unified Physics." http://academy.resonance.is/topic/4-2-2 -99-9999999999996-space. Accessed July 15, 2015.

Schneider, Michael S. *A Beginner's Guide to Constructing the Universe: The Mathematical Archetypes of Nature, Art, and Science.* New York: HarperCollins Publishers, 1994.

Schwaller de Lubicz, René Adolphe. *Sacred Science: The King of Pharaonic Theocracy.* Translated by André and Goldian VandenBroeck. Rochester, Vt.: Inner Traditions International, 1988.

———. *The Temple in Man: Sacred Architecture and the Perfect Man.* Translated by Robert and Deborah Lawlor. New York: Inner Traditions International, 1977.

SciTechDaily. "Atomic Bond Types Clearly Discernible Thanks to Single-Molecule Images." *Science and Technology News,* 2012. http://scitechdaily .com/atomic-bond-types-clearly-discernible-thanks-to-single-molecule -images. Accessed February 3, 2015.

Scott, Jeff. "Birds, Thermals, and Soaring Flight." AeroWeb. Retrieved from www .aerospaceweb.org/question/nature/q0253.shtml, 2005. Accessed June 15, 2015.

Scranton, Laird. *China's Cosmological Prehistory: The Sophisticated Science Encoded in Civilization's Earliest Symbols.* Rochester, Vt.: Inner Traditions, 2014.

———. *The Cosmological Origins of Myth and Symbol: From the Dogon and Ancient Egypt to India, Tibet, and China.* Rochester, Vt.: Inner Traditions, 2010.

Seawright, Carolyn. "Egypt: Amentet, Goddess of the Dead, Personification of the West." www.touregypt.net/featurestories/amentet.htm. Accessed June 30, 2015.

Shah, Nadiya. *Astrology Realized: Your Journey to Understanding Astrology.* Synchronicity Publications. 2013. https://read.amazon.com/?asin =B00BH8OLRC.

Snow Crystals. "Snowflake Branching: The Origin of the Complex Structure of Snowflakes." www.its.caltech.edu/~atomic/snowcrystals/dendrites/dendrite .htm, 1999. Accessed February 1, 2015.

Sitchin, Zecharia. *Genesis Revisited.* New York: Avon Books, 1990.

Stewart, Ian. *The Mathematics of Life.* New York: Basic Books, 2011.

Strehlow, Wighard, and Gottfried Hertzka. *Hildegard of Bingen's Medicine.* Rochester, Vt.: Bear and Company, Inc., 1988.

Suddath, Ralph. "Vibration, Energy, and Water." *ExtraOrdinary Technology* 3 (4), n.d.

Tarnas, Richard. *Cosmos and Psyche: Imitations of a New World View.* New York: Plume, 2007.

Teia, Luis. 2016. "Ancient Babylonian Use of the Pythagorean Theorem and its Three Dimensions." www.ancient-origins.net/human-origins-science

/ancient-babylonian-use-pythagorean-theorem-and-its-three-dimensions
-005199?nopaging=1. Last modified January 19, 2016.

Tellinger, Michael. *Slave Species of the Gods: The Secret History of the Anunnaki and Their Mission on Earth.* Rochester, Vt.: Bear and Company, 2012.

——. *African Temples of the Anunnaki: The Lost Technologies of the Gold Mines of Enki.* Rochester, Vt.: Bear and Company, 2013.

Theon of Smyrna. *Mathematics Useful for Understanding Plato.* Translated by Robert Lawlor and Deborah Lawlor. San Diego, Calif.: Wizards Bookshelf, 1979.

Today in Science. "Johannes Kepler's Quotations." www.todayinsci.com/K /Kepler_Johannes/KeplerJohannes-Quotations.html. Accessed February 10, 2015.

Tompkins, Peter, and Christopher Bird. *The Secret Life of Plants: A Fascinating Account of the Physical, Emotional, and Spiritual Relations between Plants and Man.* New York: HarperCollins Publishers, 1973.

Vaid, Vashisht. *Brahmandic Gyanum: Universal Knowledge.* N.p.: The Divine Vision, 2012.

——. *The Secrets of Astrology.* N.p.: The Global Movement, 2012.

Veggi, Athon, and Alison Davidson. *The Book of Doors Divination Deck: An Alchemical Oracle from Ancient Egypt.* Rochester, Vt.: Destiny Books, 1995.

Wasserman, James. *Art and Symbols of the Occult, Images of Power and Wisdom.* Rochester, Vt.: Destiny Books, 1993.

Watson, A. and J. Lovelock. *Biological Homeostasis of the Global Environment: The Parable of Daisyworld.* N.p.: Tellus, 1983.

West, John Anthony. *Serpent in the Sky: The High Wisdom of Ancient Egypt.* Wheaton, Ill.: Quest Books, 1993.

Wilcock, David. *The Hidden Science of Lost Civilisations: The Source Field Investigations.* London: Souvenir Press, 2012.

Wilhelm, Richard, trans. *The Secret of the Golden Flower: A Chinese Book of Life.* San Diego: Harcourt Brace and Company, 1962.

Wilhelm, Richard, and Cary F. Baynes. *The I Ching, or Book of Changes.* Princeton: Princeton University Press, 1977.

Willner, John. *The Perfect Horoscope.* New York: Paraview Press, 2001.

Wong, Eva. *Tales of the Dancing Dragon: Stories of the Tao.* Boston: Shambhala Publications, Inc., 2007.

INDEX